SARS-CoV2 (COVID-19) Pandemic Control and Prevention

This is the first comprehensive text to provide not only a detailed explanation of how the SARS-CoV2 (COVID-19) virus is spread within human populations, but also an epidemiological analysis and interpretation of viral pandemics to enable better measures for prevention and control.

Providing an introduction to the physiology of both the human immune system and the SARS-CoV2 virus, specifically the virus's replicative potential and our own vulnerability, the book offers an in-depth understanding of how the pandemic evolved. It also highlights the aberrant epigenomic mechanistic process in pathogenic microbes' replication and survival, implying gene and environment interaction that affected different populations. Citing a range of environmental conditions, from structural and systemic racism to malnutrition and low-socioeconomic status, the book examines how these factors exacerbated existing health disparities, resulting in a disproportionate burden of morbidity and mortality on certain social groups.

Also providing invaluable guidance on how future iterations of this pandemic may be better prevented and controlled, this will be a defining book for students, researchers and professionals within Public Health and Clinical Medicine to better understand the SARS-CoV2 (COVID-19) virus, and how to protect the most vulnerable social groups.

Laurens (Larry) Holmes, Jr is an immunologist and infectious disease specialist, and obtained an additional doctoral degree in cancer epidemiology and biostatistics from the University of Texas, Health Sciences Center at Houston. He is a Principal Translational Research Scientist, a former Founding Director of the Nemours Paediatric Translational Health Disparities Science Research, Training and Education Program, Wilmington, DE (USA), a leading proponent of epigenomic epidemiology in clinical medicine and public health and Affiliate professor of molecular epidemiology and clinical trials at the Biological Sciences Department at the University of Delaware, Newark, DE (USA), Co-founder and Director of Global Health Equity Foundation (GHEF-USA) and Founding Director of Lawhols International Scientific Research Consulting, LIS-RC (USA). Professor Holmes is currently a Director of the Graduate Public Health Program (Epidemiology and Global Health), Public Health & Allied Health Sciences Department, Wesley College-Delaware State University, Dover, DE (USA).

SARS-CoV2 (COVID-19) Pandemic Control and Prevention

An Epidemiological Perspective

Laurens Holmes, Jr

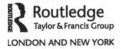

Routledge
Taylor & Francis Group

LONDON AND NEW YORK

First published 2024
by Routledge
4 Park Square, Milton Park, Abingdon, Oxon OX14 4RN

and by Routledge
605 Third Avenue, New York, NY 10158

Routledge is an imprint of the Taylor & Francis Group, an informa business

British Library Cataloguing-in-Publication Data
A catalogue record for this book is available from the British Library

Library of Congress Cataloging-in-Publication Data
Names: Holmes, Larry, Jr., 1960– author.
Title: SARS-CoV2 (COVID-19) pandemic control and prevention: an epidemiological perspective / Laurens Holmes, Jr.
Description: Abingdon, Oxon: New York, NY: Routledge, 2024. |
Includes bibliographical references and index. |
Identifiers: LCCN 2023016327 | ISBN 9781032543543 (hardback) |
ISBN 9781032543550 (paperback) | ISBN 9781003424451 (ebook)
Subjects: MESH: COVID-19—epidemiology | SARS-CoV-2—physiology |
COVID-19—prevention & control | COVID-19 Vaccines | Socioeconomic
Disparities in Health
Classification: LCC RA644.C67 | NLM WC 506.41 |
DDC 614.5/924144—dc23/eng/20230703
LC record available at https://lccn.loc.gov/2023016327

ISBN: 978-1-032-54354-3 (hbk)
ISBN: 978-1-032-54355-0 (pbk)
ISBN: 978-1-003-42445-1 (ebk)

DOI: 10.4324/9781003424451

Typeset in Times New Roman
by codeMantra

Dedicated to

Colin Powell, First Black/AA Secretary of State (in memoriam) due to COVID-19 complications and multiple myeloma.

Palmer Beasley, MD, MPH, former Dean and Professor emeritus, University of Texas –School of Public Health (in memoriam), who dedicated his career to the evaluation of chronic hepatic disease in hepatocellular carcinoma.

James Steele, DVM, MPH, retired US Assistant Surgeon General, Professor emeritus, University of Texas – School of Public Health (in memoriam), who dedicated his career to improving public health, especially among racial/ethnic minorities.

Mom, **KMIA** (in memoriam), Grandma, **NUA,** (in memoriam) Dad, **Morrison Holmes** (in memoriam) and Grandad, **Duke Holmes** (in memoriam) who dedicated their lives to ensuring that children and families in need were provided with basic needs (health, food and shelter).

Contents

Preface

"SARS-CoV2 survivability depends on how we as the human society apply dynamic and reliable data on predisposing risk factors in control and preventive measures."

—**Laurens Holmes, Jr**

Global pandemics reflect the colonization of pathogenic microbes, due in part to the limited scientific knowledge in ensuring marginalized transmissibility, severity, case fatality and mortality, as observed in SARS-CoV2, the causative pathogen in the COVID-19 pandemic. The application of reliable, accurate and valid information regarding viral incubation period, transmission mode, clinical manifestations, complications and survival allows for pandemic mitigation and ultimate regression to the SARS-CoV2 pre-pandemic era. However, pandemic control and preventive measures remain transitional, given uncertainties in scientific evidence discovery, implying the random error quantification prior to the findings generalizability and application in SARS-CoV2 transmission mitigation and COVID-19 marginalized severity, hospitalization, prognosis and mortality. Despite the observed direction, pathogenic microbes or viral spread, severity and mortality fundamentally implicates environmental variance in the observed clinical outcomes and subpopulation differentials.

The knowledge and application of the core functions of public health, namely assessment, policy and assurance, are vital to national and global pandemic mitigation and marginalization initiatives. Since public health reflects what we as a society do to remain healthy, human populations need to ensure that the goal of public health is utilized in pandemic control, implying disease control and health promotion practices. While the United States Center for Disease Control and Prevention (CDC) and the World Health Organization recommends the application of what is known about this pandemic in enhancing community herd immunity through vaccine uptake for the vaccine eligible, there remains vaccine hesitancy, adversely impacting SARS-CoV2 community herd immunity, providing this pathogen the opportunity for mutation. Further, the allocation of resources and vaccines to under-developed nations as well as the resources for these administrations remain a pathway to COVID-19 pandemic mitigation and novel variants margination, since we all live in a global village.

This book utilizes a simplified and reliable approach in describing **SARS-CoV2** as the coronavirus initially associated with South Asia Respiratory Syndrome 1 (2003), prior to this **COVID-19 (Co = corona; Vi = virus, D = disease, 19 = 2019)** global pandemic caused by SARS-CoV2, implying **South Asia Respiratory Syndrome 2 (SARS-CoV2)**. This pathogen, SARS-CoV2, first emerged in Wuhan, China in November 2019. The microbiologic characterization of this pathogenic microbe is described, which allows for the understanding of the immunologic concept of antigenicity, epitope and antibodies generation as well as immune system integration, with respect to immune system responsiveness.

SARS-CoV2 is a corona virus with 79% genome sequence compared to SARS-CoV and 50% compared with MERS-CoV. There are six functional open reading frames (ORFs) arranged in order from 5′ to 3′: replicase (ORF1a/ORF1b), spike (S), envelope (E), membrane (M) and nucleocapsid (N). There are seven putative ORFs encoding accessory proteins and are interspersed between the structural genes25. The majority of the proteins encoded by SARS-CoV2 have a similar length to the corresponding proteins in SARS-CoV. Within the four structural genes, SARS-CoV2 shares an estimated 90% amino acid (AA) with SARS-CoV except for SARS-CoV2 S gene with differential.

With the limited knowledge of SARS-CoV2 incubation period, transmission mode and sero-positivity, this book basically explains these dimensions. The risk and predisposing factors are observed in several chapters implying, though not limited to, social determinants of health and socio-demographics. For example, the following risk and predisposing factors in SARS-CoV2 transmissibility were observed: population density, age, race, sex, gender, ethnicity, comorbidities, pregnancy, socioeconomic status, geographic locale, seasonality, etc.

The subpopulation variances or disparities in case positivity, severity, case fatality and mortality in SARS-CoV2 and COVID-19 are explained, with racial/ethnic minorities described or observed with this disproportionate burden of SARS-CoV2 pandemic. With such observation, this literature recommends the application of disproportionate universalism in the timely allocation of health resources to racial and ethnic minorities in future pandemics. While pathogenic microbes require the host cell for survival, implying replications and mutagenic initiative, human hosts are responsible in the mitigation and marginalization of this SARS-CoV2 initiative. This book very clearly explains the role of immunization in community herd immunity enhancement and recommends all vaccine-eligible humans to be fully vaccinated. Additionally, vaccine hesitancy is cautioned in this literature since hesitancy reflects ignorance of the benefits of vaccines in all settings, although not absolute since individuals with malignant neoplasm, especially hematologic and multiple myeloma, are less likely to fully generate antibodies following vaccine uptake.

SARS-CoV2 (COVID-19) Pandemic Control and Prevention: An Epidemiological Perspective reflects translational scientific information in current and future pandemic stabilization and spread mitigation. This book comprises three sections: (A) SARS-CoV2 Basic Immune System Responsiveness and Descriptive Epidemiology; (B) SARS-CoV2 Qualitative Systematic Review (QSR) and Qualitative Evidence Synthesis (QualES) and (C) SARS-CoV2 Inferential and Quantitative Epidemiologic Approach. Section A explains the structure and the function of the immune system and well as viral pathogenic microbes with specific focus on SARS-CoV2. This section applies a non-inferential approach as descriptive in the understanding of the prevalence and cumulative incidence of SARS-CoV2 and COVID-19 predisposing factors and risk in transmission and infectivity as well as case fatality and mortality. Section B applies the qualitative systematic review and QualES in summary findings, thus facilitating recommendations for SARS-CoV2 prevention and control. Section C applies pre-existing data as cross-sectional ecologic, as well as reliable scientific evidence discovery methodology in subpopulation risk differentials in SARS-CoV2 transmissibility and COVID-19 clinical manifestations, severity, comorbidities, case fatality, prognosis and mortality.

Since scientific evidence is by no means an individual effort, but transdisciplinary, translational and team science as observed by the author, Professor Laurens Holmes, Jr, this book applies this dimension in recommending a translational and transdisciplinary approach in adherence to control and preventive measures in this pandemic. Additionally, since scientific information remains translational and dynamic, readers are required to reflect on the information within this book, as well as comparable data prior to decision making in applied public health settings.

However, as epidemiology like medicine remains an imprecise and inexact science, readers are encouraged to consult with other reliable and accurate sources for the information herein, and the application of these data for intervention mapping (disease control and prevention) in preventing future pandemics, thus enhancing community herd immunity. Finally, given the author of this book is a major proponent of epigenomic medicine and public health, this book recommends the evaluation of gene and environment interaction, termed aberrant epigenomic modulations in viral mitigation, vaccine effectiveness and durability in future pandemics.

Acknowledgements

"Evidence discovery and application depends on team science, transdisciplinary and translational (3 Ts) initiative, requiring scientific collegiality, as well as mutualistic, symbiotic and dynamic direction."

—*Laurens Holmes, Jr*
Medical College of Wisconsin,
Health Disparities Measures Seminar,
Podcast, 2017

Scientific knowledge remains dynamic and not static in clinical and public health decision making. This approach requires time and dedication in balancing dynamic and static data for viral pathogens control and prevention as observed in SARS-CoV2, a causative pathogen in COVID-19.

The initiation of this book reflects interest and dedication of the fellows from a Translational Health Disparities Research Program, who contributed to the publication of one of the initial works on COVID-19 Black-White case fatality and mortality differentials early in the pandemic. This publication motivated the preparation of this book that allows for the understanding of the underlying causes of the disproportionate burden of SARS-CoV2 seropositivity and COVID-19 mortality among Blacks/African Americans, Hispanics/Latino and American Indians/Alaska Natives in the US.

One is extremely grateful to all those who facilitated some of the changes and modifications, in enhancing the readability of the information in this book, namely Dr. D. Ogungbade, Dr. Prachi Carvan, Dr. Valecia John, Dr. Tatina Picolli, Dr. Doriel Ward, Dr. Monica Garrison, Dr. Aidina Williams, Dr. Maura Poleon, Jannaile Williams, MPH, PhD(c), Dr. Pascal Ngalim, Dr. Fancis Kate, Bejamin Ogundele, MPH, Dr. Michael Enwere, Kume Nsongka, MHA etc.

Professor (Dr) Holmes, wishes to thank his entire family, Maddy, Kenzie, Landon, Devin, Aiden, Anne, Victor, Julie, Brian, Paul, Dr. Ene Abi, Thomas, Charles, Victor II, Fidelis, Elizabeth, Paula, Faith St. Rose, Quan St. Rose, Dr. Glen Philipcien etc. for the time away from them during the preparation of this book. Immense thanks for all those who encouraged and motivated me.

Finally, thanks to Dr. Kerti Deepika for her passion and encouragement in assisting with the review of this book. Additionally, thanks are due to her son who provided her with time to work in assisting this book for typos and format.

Laurens Holmes, Jr

Scientific Uncertainties

Epidemiology as an applied science in public health and clinical medicine with primary focus on disease and health-related events distribution and determinants at a specific population level, remains an ever-changing discipline and profession. The author has consulted with various scientific information sources, ascertained to be reliable in the presentation of these materials on SARS-CoV2 transmission, clinical manifestations, case-fatality, survival and mortality as a translational epidemiologic perspective. However, due to the possibility of human errors and the emergence of new data on this pathogenic microbe, SARS-CoV2, a causative pathogen in COVID-19 clinical condition, the author or publisher are not responsible for any error arising from the use of these materials in future viral pandemic epidemic curve flattening, stabilization and marginalization. Therefore, readers are advised to consult with similar texts, should such texts exist, in this SARS-CoV2 Control and Preventive Measures, Translational Epidemiologic Perspective for the confirmation of information herein.

Laurens Holmes, Jr

Figures

Tables

Explanation of Sections

SECTION A - Chapters 1-17

Immune System Responsiveness, Epidemiologic Methods and Descriptive Epidemiology:
SARS-CoV2 (COVID-19)

Scientific evidence discovery is by no means an individual effort, and without team science and transdisciplinary initiatives, evidence is prone to incompleteness, uncertainties and limitations. This section explains the basic function of the human immune system and the implication of viral agents, namely pathogenic microbes as non-self in human innate and adaptive immune responsiveness. With SARS-CoV2 as a pathogenic microbe, implying the host response upon transmission, the appropriate response with respect to non-specific or innate, such as neutrophils and macrophages as well as the adaptive and specific immune response by the immunoglobulin and Helper T-cells (CD4) marginalizes viral replication, implying no clinical manifestations. However if the immune system remains unresponsive, SARS-CoV2 initiates replication and elaboration, resulting in clinical manifestations, severity and mortality.

Further, if the immunization rates in the population with pandemic increases, > 80%, implying community herd immunity enhancement, SARS-CoV2 transmission stabilizes and marginalized, resulting in viral variants, or mutations inhibition and eradication. The descriptive epidemiology provides the understanding of the distribution of SARS-CoV2 as well as the risk and predisposing factors as determinants at the specific population level. Additionally this approach allows the understanding of the pathway in risk reduction based on the specific populations' SARS-CoV2 incidence and prevalence differentials in infectivity as sero-positivity, case fatality, and mortality

SECTION B - Chapters 18–24

Qualitative Systematic Review (QSR) and Qualitative Evidence Synthesis (QualES) – SARS-
CoV2 & COIVID-19

This section applies a literature review as a qualitative systematic review (QSR) as well as a novel review methodology termed Qualitative Evidence Synthesis (QualES). The current QualES approach involves the review of published literature on SARS-CoV2 and COVID-19 risk and predisposing factors, subpopulations incidence and prevalence, prognosis and mortality. The QSR and QualES involves the utilization of a reliable online search engine such as PubMed with accurate search terms in identifying reliable scientific manuscript based of the quality criteria of the published literature. With the strategy that meets eligibility and ineligibility prior to the synopsis and synthesis as summary of the findings, this QRS and QualES remain a reliable pathway in SARS-CoV2 and COVID-19 control and prevention in meeting the public health goals in pandemic stabilization, curve flattening, case fatality and mortality marginalization, nationally and globally.

Design: A systematic review as a qualitative evidence synthesis (QualES) was used to examine the SARS-CoV2 and COVID-19 subpopulations prevalence, risk and predisposing factors as well as control and preventive measures. This research methodology implies the utilization of published literature in addressing the research question. A review of literature without a quantitative initiative was used in addressing this questions. The utilized approach allows for the synopsis based on how preventive and control measures marginalizes SARS-CoV2 spread and mortality. Since this literature review is not a quantitative systematic review, there was no application of Meta-Analysis, implying either a fixed or random effect method in this evidence discovery with respect to combined effect size as pool estimate and the confidence interval (CI) as well as random error quantification (p value).

Search Engine/Terms: The pubmed was used to identify published literature while basic search terms were used to extract the studies of interest based on the research questions.

Eligibility/Quality criteria: Studies with accurate and reliable objectives, research questions, variables measurement scales, analysis and outcome measures as well as reasonable sample size were utilized in this review. This approach required the assessment of most studies derived from the search engine, pubmed using the above mentioned research criteria for studies eligibility for scientific publication. Studies with sample size or case report were not included in this QualES.

Study Population, Materials & Synthesis: The study population needs to be observed. The application of QualES requires the study of study and the assessment of these studies for internal and external validity prior to the QualES design. Further, the studies utilized in this QualES were examined based on objectives, research questions, hypotheses, aims, design, analysis and reliable interpretation of the outputs as data in the tables.

SECTION C – Chapters 25–28

Analytic Epidemiologic Perspective – SARS-CoV2 & COVID-19 Pandemic

This section applies a specific epidemiologic design namely a cross-sectional-ecologic design, as an "aggregate snap shot cohort", implying a non-experimental epidemiologic approach, involving simultaneous data collection or acquisition on the exposure/independent or predictor variable, and the outcome/dependent or response variable. The scientific research strategy required the utilization of the SARS-CoV2 data at aggregate level in the statistical modeling by either logistic regression model, or binomial regression model, analyses, output tabulation, data interpretation, supported with data as result, discussion, limitations, inference as conclusion and recommendations. With respect to conclusion, since no findings are certain but driven by some uncertainties, implying the utilization of the random error quantification as p value in inference, all findings in this section, C are driven by uncertainties. However if the random error quantification is > 0.05 (5% type I error tolerance, a clinically and biologically meaningful difference of 10% is applied in the recommendation of the findings in these studies for suggestions and further studies.

This section involves an analytic or quantitative epidemiologic approach in evidence discovery in utilizing the observed findings in future intervention mapping in marginalizing and stabilizing viral pandemics. Epidemiologic designs require : (a) study conceptualization, implying a reliable research question based on PEICO (population, exposure, intervention, control/ comparison and outcome, (b) Specific aims and hypothesis, (c) study objectives, (d) specific experimental or non-experimental epidemiologic design, (e) Conduct, data collection and processing, (f) statistical analysis and output data tabulation, (g) Data interpretation as findings or results, (h) discussion of the findings from the study based on previous studies and possible explanation of the observed finding without previous studies, (i) limitations, inference as study summary or conclusion, (j) recommendations for future research approach and (k) References as citation or cited literature in support of the current study.

Analytic Epidemiologic Research Structure

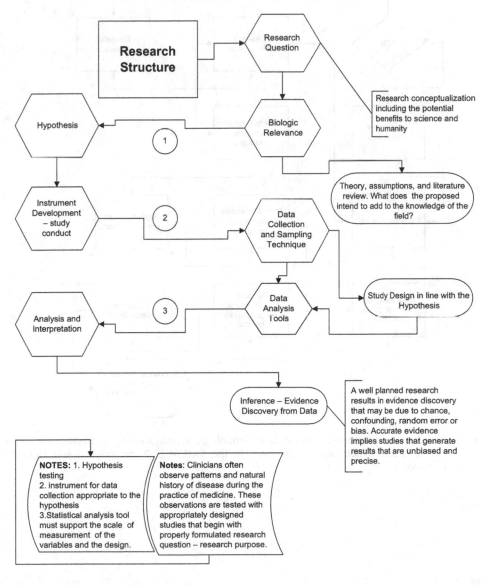

Figure I Illustrates the approach in scientific evidence discovery, implying inference as external validity.

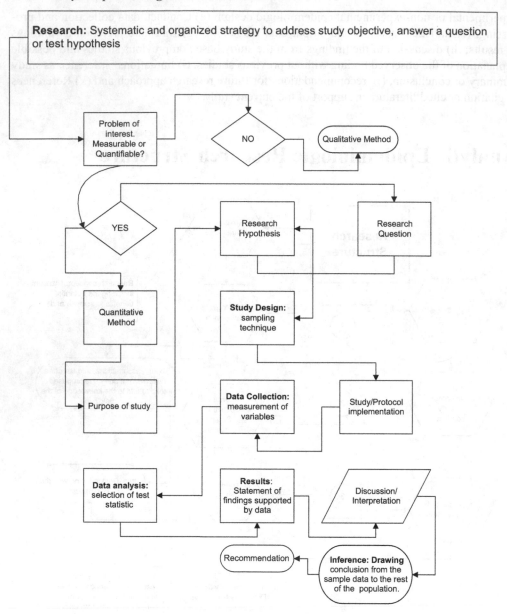

Figure II describes the quantitative method in epidemiologic investigation by addressing the research questions and hypotheses as illustrated in the SARS-CoV2 transmission and COVID-19 mortality

1 Immuno-Epidemiologic Perspective in Pathogenic Microbes

Immune System Response and Integration

Human Immune System Structure and Function

The immune system functions normally by providing a beneficial, protective function to the host. The primary function of the normal immune system, that results in this protective function, involves the ability of the cells of the immune system to differentiate self and non-self and reacts towards the non-self as an antigen.[1,2] However, in some circumstances, overreaction by this beneficial function can result in cellular damage, and even death, in a condition termed hypersensitivity reaction as in anaphylaxis and autoimmune disorders (systemic lupus and Graves' disease).[3,4]

Immune System Responsiveness: Self versus Non-Self

The basic function of the immune system is to protect the host self against antigen as non-self, by the application of a non-adaptive or non-specific response via phagocytosis, implying neutrophils interaction with antigen as well as an adaptive or specific immune response via the helper T-cells (CD4) elaboration, thanks to the macrophage implication as an antigen presenting cells (APC) prior to the CD4 cells activation and elaboration, as well as B-cells growth factors, cytokines, leukotrienes (IL) and immunoglobulin elaboration.

(1) When the normal immune system comes in contact with the self, tolerance occurs and there is no immune responsiveness. Clinical tolerance to non-self may occur in immunodeficiency due to the suppression of the immune response in conditions such as X-linked agammaglobulinemia, DiGeorge syndrome, Wiskott–Aldrich syndrome, Ataxia telangiectasia etc.[5] as well as immunosuppressant agents (radiation and chemotherapy).

(2) The presence of an antigen as non-self induces immunogenicity, implying total antigenic capacity, while haptens are partial antigens that require a carrier protein model to become immunogenic (6). A classic example of antigen reflect pathogenic microbes such as bacteria, viruses, toxins, etc.

(3) The immune system responsiveness as specific/ adaptive involves the innate/and non-adaptive cell as macrophage binding to viral pathogen as a cell such, as SARS-CoV2, and the binding of this with the MHC-I molecule, resulting in Antigen-MHC complex elaboration, leading to mitosis and the release of cytokine such as IL-4, IL-8, IL-10 on the infected cell of the human host, resulting in cell death. The integration of macrophage, T-cell and NK-cell results in less replication of SARS-CoV2.

DOI: 10.4324/9781003424451-1

(4) The IMMUNOCOMPETENT CELLS as non-adaptive and adaptive participate in the response to antigens. The specific and adaptive response is characterized by antibody namely immunoglobulin elaboration and the binding of the antigenic sites such as epitopes to the antigenic site of the immunoglobulin (B-cell). The immunocompetent cells primarily include B-CELLS (3), T-CELLS (4), NATURAL KILLER CELLS (NK-cells) (5) and LEUKOCYTES (6). The macrophage (7) represents a non-specific and non-adaptive response and facilitates the activation of CD4, as T-cell for interleukins as cytokines elaboration, as well as the BCGF (B-Cells Growth Factor) for plasma cells elaboration and immunoglobulins such as IgG, IgM, sIgA, etc. Depending on the particular response, these cells work in varied combinations to eliminate the presented antigen or foreign particles as non-self.[6]

The specific recognition of pathogenic microbe is due to proteins on the surface of the host cells. The major histocompatibility complex (MHC), also known as the human leukocyte antigen (HLA) system, is a large genomic region on human chromosome 6 that codes for these proteins. These proteins present cells to the T-cell receptor (TCR) located on the T-cell surface. The human T-cells "learn" this recognition during its development in the thymus. The B-cells are capable of independently making this determination without APC prior to its elaboration.[7]

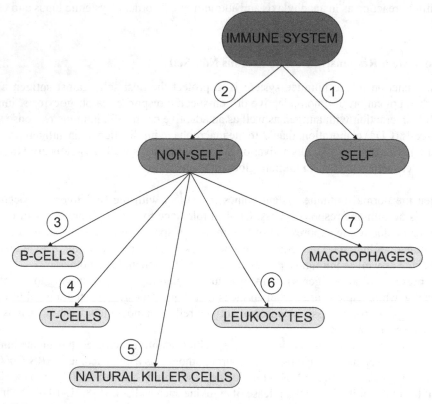

Figure 1.1. Immune System Response: Antigen as Non-Self

Note: The immune system classified as (a) SELF and (b) NON-SELF, where non-self is SARS-CoV2, requiring the host response.

Innate and Specific Immune Response: Basic Understanding

The immune response offered by the host to a foreign particle involves two fundamental divisions of the immune system, namely the natural, innate or non-specific and the acquired, adaptive or specific immune mechanistic process.

(1) The natural immune response involves normal biologic mechanisms that function without prior exposure to the antigens or microorganisms. Specifically, what the innate immunity offers to the host is a nonspecific response conferred since birth. Natural immunity is offered by several mechanisms such as anatomic, physiologic, phagocytic and inflammatory response in nature.[8]

   The immune system is traditionally classified as a non-adaptive and is indicative of instant elaboration of fever as a cardinal sign of an inflammation, epithelial cells, dendritic cells, macrophages, neutrophils and the complement components. The adaptive response requires the elaboration of B-cells, T-cells in inhibiting the SARS-CoV2 replication.

(2) The ACQUIRED (ADAPTIVE), adaptive or specific immune mechanism or response occurs following an antigenic challenge, given a non-self or foreign particle. This response is differentiated from the innate, non-adaptive or non-specific response based on the memory activation and occurrence from adaptive and specific immune responsiveness. For example, if a pathogen infects a host, the B-cell elaborates immunoglobulin G (IgG), and if the same pathogen re-infects the same host, the memory IgG neutralizes the pathogen, resulting in immune complex activation and pathogenic destruction. Simply, once an initial exposure to an antigen has occurred, the immune system exhibits this "memory". In effect, the subsequent challenges by these specific antigens as re-infection results in an enhanced immune responsiveness. Both the acquired and innate systems collaborate, by stimulating or regulating the other, in a joint effort to enhance the protection of the host as "self" from foreign particle, antigen or pathogen as "non-self".

(3–4) The ACQUIRED immune mechanism consists of two fundamental components, namely humoral and T-Cell. The humoral response is primarily mediated by the B-CELLS, and the cell-mediated response primarily involves the activated T-CELLS. These two responses may occur independently or simultaneously.

   The adaptive, specific and non-innate immune response requires antigen binding to the dendritic cell and the binding to naïve T-cell, resulting in the activation of this cell and the T-cell replication. This process results in the T-cell differentiation, resulting in cytokines elaboration such as IL-4 and IL-2, enhancing phagocytes, T-killer and B-cells elaboration as immune cells activation.

(5) The anatomic barriers are mechanical barriers that directly prevent the entry or procession of invading pathogens.[9] The main anatomic barrier is the intact skin. The conjunctivae, alimentary, respiratory and urogenital tracts are protected by mucous membranes. Furthermore, saliva, tears, urine and mucous secretions act to trap and wash away microorganisms or pathogenic microbes from the host. Finally, ciliary apparatus that line the respiratory tract prevent the forward progression of pathogens, and propel pathogens trapped in mucous outward in a synchronous motion.

(6) The physiologic barriers mediate pathogens via thermal, chemical or pneumatic inhibition. Normal body temperature is unsuitable for some pathogens to thrive in. Fever

produced by endogenous pyrogens (such as IL-1, elaborated from macrophages and monocytes), and exogenous pyrogens further inhibit some pathogen proliferation, and can intensify the activity of interferons.[10] Gastrointestinal pH and digestive enzymes create an acidic environment, destroying and inhibiting the multiplication and colonization of most ingested microorganisms. The acidic nature of the vagina also renders such protection, with the pH value (0–14) of the vaginal mucosa <7 (acidity). Other chemical components include lysozyme in mucous secretions and tears (hydrolyze peptidoglycan in bacterial cell walls), lactic and fatty acids in the sebum (maintain skin pH of 3–5), complement in plasma (when activated, destroy pathogens), interferons (antiviral activity) and collectins (surfactant that disrupts lipid membranes). Additionally, O_2 (Oxygen) tension can prevent the multiplication of anaerobic pathogens.

(7) The INFLAMMATORY response results in enhanced phagocytosis, through the steps of vasodilation, increased capillary permeability, and the resultant efflux of phagocytes from the capillaries into the injured tissue. Chemical mediators of inflammation include acute-phase proteins such as C-reactive protein, which activates the complement system. The histamine is involved in the vasodilation and increased permeability described above.[11] Inactivated plasma kinins are activated by injury and have the same basic effect as histamines, implying increased vascular permeability and vasodilation.

(8) The PHAGOCYTIC processes include destruction of extracellular material by phagocytosis, a form of endocytosis in which foreign particulate matter is engulfed, and other endocytotic processes such as pinocytosis, [12] implying uptake of fluid.

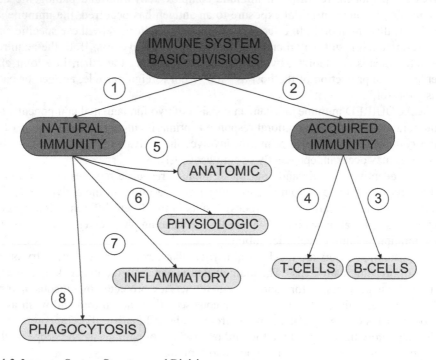

Figure 1.2 Immune System Structure and Division

Note: Natural as non-adaptive and non-specific; while acquired is characterized as adaptive and specific immune response.

Acquired or Specific Immune Response

The acquired immune response is characterized by two responses, namely cell-mediated and humoral. The cell-mediated immune response is associated with the activated T-cells, while the humoral immune response is regulated by the B-cells, and includes a primary and complement component. The acquired and specific responses involving the antibody (immunoglobulin) and the T-cells are characterized by specificity and memory, implying increased response by effector molecules following a re-infection with the same pathogenic microbe.[13] The cells of the lymphoid lineage (B- and T-lymphocytes) of the immune response offer an acquired response to the host. Below is Figure 1.3 on the cell-mediated and humoral immune response.

(1) The CELL-MEDIATED RESPONSE, though a misnomer, reflects the immune response primarily offered by the T-cells. The T-cell response involves the MHC-I, and the utilization of antigen presenting cells (APC) such as macrophage and the binding of the IL=1 receptor resulting in further interleukins as cytokines elaboration.

(2) The HUMORAL IMMUNE RESPONSE involves the extracellular fluids such as serum and lymph, primarily refers to antibody response involving the plasma cells and the B-cells.

(3) The SPECIFIC HUMORAL immune system refers to the B-cell antibody defense, a flexible adaptor molecule with a series of different surface shapes, which enable it to bind to the surface of different microbes, hence specific reactivity. The antibody can also bind to phagocytic cells through its Fc fragment, thus enhancing phagocytosis by opsonization.

(4) The IMMUNOGLOBULINS (antibodies) are generated following the B-cell activation to plasma cells. The immunoglobulins offer adaptive, humoral and specific immune responses.

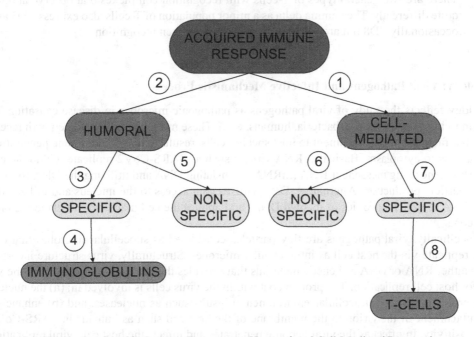

Figure 1.3 Acquired or Specific Immune Response as Humoral and Cell-Mediated Responsiveness

Note: The acquired response is classified as humoral and cell-mediated. Humoral immune response required immunoglobulin as antibodies, while cell-mediated reflects the T-cells.

(5) The NON-SPECIFIC HUMORAL (COMPLEMENT SYSTEM) immune response refers to the activation of the complement system. The commencement of the complement system activation involves the complement system component, C3, and the binding of this component with the immune complex (antibody-antigen). Specifically, immunology often classifies the complement system as part of the innate immune system, as non-adaptive or specific in nature. However, the classical pathway of complement system activation often results from the aggregation of antibodies such as IgM and IgG. Following activation, cleavage products act as opsonin and chemotaxis, enhancing or facilitating phagocytosis. Therefore, the complement system must be taken into consideration when discussing acquired immunity, as it could be activated by the immunoglobulins-antigen complex.

(6) The NON-SPECIFIC CELL-MEDIATED immune response is offered by the phagocytic cells such as the macrophages, neutrophils and monocytes. This defense involves the engulfment, digestion and destruction of microbes or foreign particles. While some texts refer to phagocytosis and the molecules involved as strictly innate, it must be taken into consideration that macrophages are involved in antigen presentation to the T-cells. Furthermore, phagocytic cells, while not specific for antigen, can bind antibodies via their Fc receptors, with resultant lysis of the target, termed antibody-dependent cell-mediated cytotoxicity (ADCC).

(7–8) The SPECIFIC CELL-MEDIATED immune response is offered by the T-cells, with development beginning in the bone marrow, then migration to the thymus where differentiation takes place resulting in functional T-cell production. The thymic differentiation begins in the cortex, eventually yielding CD4+CD8+ (double positive), and then proceeds to the medulla with resultant CD4+CD8− and CD4−CD8+ (single positives). There are two general types of T-cells with recognition complexes that observe antigen quite differently. The gamma delta as a minor population of T-cells also express CD3 and occasionally CD8 but are not MHC restricted in antigen recognition.

Virology: Viral Pathogens and Infective Mechanistic Process

Virology reflects the study of viral pathogens as pathogenic microbes in disease causation involving viruses and the host (bacteria, humans, etc.). These microbes are associated with receptors that facilitate their attachment to host specific cells, resulting in cell membrane penetration and access to cytoplasm. Basically, RNA viruses such as SARS-CoV2 replicate within the cytoplasm, generating messenger RNA (mRNA), translating DNA and utilizing the DNA for new virus particle production. Alternately, DNA viruses gain access to the nucleus and utilizes the host DNA to generate copies of its own DNA, and applies the cell machinery to elaborate protein coats.[14]

Specifically, viral pathogens are tiny particles considered as subcellular microbes that can only replicate via the host cell as intra–cellular microbes. Structurally, virus structure incorporates either RNA or DNA as genetic materials that provides the information required by the virus for host cell replication. The protein coat within the virus cells is involved in: (a) the nucleic acid protection from extracellular environmental insults such as nucleases, and (b) enhancing the attachment of the virion to the membrane of the host cell such as humans in SARS-CoV2 seropositivity. In effect as the viral genome penetrates and infects the host cell, viral replication requires the human as the host cell for energy elaboration and replication. Since viruses are intracellular microbes, implying host immune system down regulation and viral protection, as well as the host cell exponential immune response in different hosts or individuals exposed to

SARS-CoV2, severity, complications and mortality varies with or without therapeutics. Simply, the host response to viral infection signals the individual's physiologic response namely swelling, hyperemia, fever, pain (inflammatory mechanistic process) and interferon elaboration for host protection.[15]

Basically, several viron parts are separately synthesized within the host cell, resulting in progeny particles formation. Significant viral genomes are very adaptable once access is gained to the cell membrane, resulting in viral replication in almost any cell within the host. Since viral survivability depends on the host cell, mild infections remain, resulting in mild to moderate infectivity, with mortality differentials. However, with respect to SARS-CoV2, the host cell undergoes symptoms severity, implying complications, renal organ damage and failure, leading to excess host mortality and viral mutation with novel strains for enhanced SARS-CoV2 transmission opportunity.[16] In addressing SARS-CoV2 transmission and host dependence, the scientific and public health communities require the assessment of virus-host dependence and the application of such data in transmissibility marginalization and COVID-19 pre-pandemic ecosystem stabilization.

Questions for Discussion

1. What is immunology? Describe the immune system and integration with other human biologic systems.
2. Suppose an individual is infected with SARS-CoV2, how could the immune system responsiveness be explained?
3. If an individual is exposed to SARS-CoV2 seropositive and is not infected, how could the host immune system be explained?
4. What is the difference between innate and adaptive immune system with respect to SARS-CoV2 infectivity?
5. Explain the role of NK-cells in viral replication downregulation as well as the NK-cell integration with T-cells and B-cells during viral replication.

Notes

1 "Overview of Immune Response During SARS-CoV-2 Infection". 7 Aug. 2020, https://www.frontiersin.org/articles/10.3389/fimmu.2020.01949/full. Accessed 9 Mar. 2022.
2 "Features, Evaluation, and Treatment of Coronavirus (COVID-19)". https://www.ncbi.nlm.nih.gov/books/NBK554776/. Accessed 9 Mar. 2022.
3 "Control of Viral Infections by Epigenetic-targeted Therapy". 27 Mar. 2019, https://clinicalepigeneticsjournal.biomedcentral.com/articles/10.1186/s13148-019-0654-9. Accessed 9 Mar. 2022.
4 "An Introduction to Immunology and Immunopathology." 12 Sep. 2018, https://aacijournal.biomedcentral.com/articles/10.1186/s13223-018-0278-1. Accessed 9 Mar. 2022.
5 "The ITP Syndrome: Pathogenic and Clinical Diversity | Blood – ASH ...". https://ashpublications.org/blood/article/113/26/6511/26188/ The-ITP-syndrome-pathogenic-and-clinical-diversity. Accessed 9 Mar. 2022.
6 "Antibody Production (Immunogen Preparation) – Thermo Fisher". https://www.thermofisher.com/in/en/home/life-science/antibodies/antibodies-learning-center/antibodies-resource-library/antibody-methods/antibody-production-immunogen-preparation.html. Accessed 9 Mar. 2022.
7 "Adaptive Immune Response – Concepts of Biology – BC Open ...". https://opentextbc.ca/biology/chapter/23-2-adaptive-immune-response/. Accessed 9 Mar. 2022.
8 "Investigating the Peptide-MHC Specificity of Alloreactive T Cells and ...". 27 Nov. 2017, https://escholarship.umassmed.edu/cgi/viewcontent.cgi?article=1948&context=gsbs_diss. Accessed 9 Mar. 2022.
9 "Immune system | Description, Function, & Facts – Encyclopedia ...". https://www.britannica.com/science/immune-system. Accessed 9 Mar. 2022.

10 "Barriers to Pathogens – Biology LibreTexts". 5 Mar. 2021, https://bio.libretexts.org/Bookshelves/Introductory_and_General_Biology/Book%3A_Introductory_Biology_(CK-12)/13%3A_Human_Biology/13.47%3A_Barriers_to_Pathogens. Accessed 9 Mar. 2022.
11 "Fever | Definition, Characteristics, & Causes – Encyclopedia Britannica". https://www.britannica.com/science/fever. Accessed 9 Mar. 2022.
12 "The Crucial Roles of Inflammatory Mediators in Inflammation: A Review". 15 May 2018, https://www.ncbi.nlm.nih.gov/pmc/articles/PMC5993766/. Accessed 9 Mar. 2022.
13 "Phagocytosis (Article) | Cells | Khan Academy". https://www.khanacademy.org/test-prep/mcat/cells/transport-across-a-cell-membrane/a/phagocytosis. Accessed 9 Mar. 2022.
14 "Adaptive Immune Response – Concepts of Biology – BC Open …". https://opentextbc.ca/biology/chapter/23-2-adaptive-immune-response/. Accessed 9 Mar. 2022.
15 "Mechanisms of Cell and Tissue Damage – NCBI". https://www.ncbi.nlm.nih.gov/pmc/articles/PMC7158287/. Accessed 9 Mar. 2022.
16 "Infectious Diseases of the Gastrointestinal Tract – NCBI". https://www.ncbi.nlm.nih.gov/pmc/articles/PMC7152230/. Accessed 9 Mar. 2022.

2 Immuno-Epidemiologic Perspective in Pathogenic Microbes
Epidemiologic Principles and Concepts

History of Epidemiology and Current Trajectory

Epidemiology remains a profession not merely a discipline, and emerges from the Greek notion of the assessment, examination or study of what is upon people. Literally, "epi" means "upon", "demos" means "people" and "logos" means study. Simply, epidemiology implies the assessment of exposure or occurrence that is beyond normal at the human population level. As the basic and applied science of public health, the role of epidemiology in disease control and prevention remains that of assessing the distribution and determinants of disease and health-related events at the specific population level and the utilization of these data in intervention mapping.[1]

Between 1978 and 2017, the term epidemiology serves as a discipline in characterizing the application of the terms, "problems", "knowledge", "public health", "population", "study", "disease", "health", and "distribution" in societal health conditions such as morbidity and mortality. With these terms, epidemiology is basically the study of disease and health-related events or phenomena such as pregnancy, well-child visits and immunization at the population level. Specifically, with this notion and the application of "science", epidemiology reflects a scientific approach in the assessment of the distribution and determinants of disease, health-related events, survival and mortality at the population level.

Epidemiology: Current Concept and Application

Although epidemiology has been given many definitions from its modern and formal inception, it remains a population health science focused primarily on the distribution and determinants of disease, injuries, disabilities, and health related events at the population level and the application of such knowledge to disease prevention and control. Epidemiology is simply a population-oriented discipline that quantifies, locates, and determines causes and mechanisms of health-related states or events and applies this knowledge to prevention and control of health-related events in specified populations. Epidemiology has traditionally been defined as the study of the distribution and determinants of health-related events in the human population and the application of this knowledge to disease, disability, and injury control and prevention. As a basic science of public health, epidemiology is involved in the assessment, surveillance and monitoring of health status at the population level and the application of these results in disease prevention and control, such as with COVID-19. Specifically, epidemiology deals with measurement of disease occurrence and frequency in the population; identification of when, where and within which population subgroups health-related events are more or less likely to occur; determining the causes at the population level; determining the mechanisms of causation, natural history and the clinical course of the health-related events; and application of the results to the prevention and control of disease and health-related events.

DOI: 10.4324/9781003424451-2

Epidemiology: Application in Clinical/Biomedical Research

Clinical and biomedical research often involve investigation into the association between variables, identification of predictors of disease, and prognosis or outcome (response), as well as the effectiveness or efficacy of treatment modalities in a specific set of patients. Epidemiology, as the basic science of public health that deals with the distribution, determinants and prevention of disease, disabilities and injuries in human populations, plays a fundamental role in design and inference in clinical/biomedical research. For example, clinical investigation into the effect of ionizing radiation on thyroid cancer in a pediatric cancer clinic may involve a retrospective cohort or case-control design. Therefore, without a sound knowledge and application of these designs and their measures of association and effect, such studies cannot be properly conducted, implying flawed design, confounding effects, effect measure modifier or interaction, and impaired generalizability.

Disease and Health-Related Event Distribution and Determinants

The term distribution implies the frequency (number, counts, percentage, prevalence) and pattern (time, place, person) of health events in a population, while determinants imply the causes, variables and factors influencing the health-related events with respect to their occurrences. This aspect of epidemiologic method involves disease- or health-related events quantification (odds ratio, relative risk, risk ratio, hazard ratio, beta coefficient).

Specific Population and Application in Disease Distribution and Determinants

Specific population implies the health of the population/people in a community setting in contrast to clinical medicine, which is concerned with the health of an individual patient. While the primary role of epidemiology is not to control or prevent health-related events, this application provides data for public health action in controlling and preventing diseases, disabilities, and injuries, such as SARS-CoV2 and COVID-19.

Epidemiologic Design: Traditional and Modern

- **Cohort studies** are traditionally classified as (a) prospective and (b) retrospective depending on the temporal relationship between the initiation of the study and the outcome (occurrence of disease or event of interest).
- A design is considered **retrospective cohort**, which is also termed historical cohort or non-concurrent prospective study, if the exposures and the outcomes of interest (disease, for example) have already occurred prior to the initiation of the study.
- In **prospective design**, the exposure, which defines the cohort, has occurred in the exposed group prior to the initiation of the study but the outcome (disease) has not occurred. In this context, both groups are followed to assess the incidence rate of the disease, comparing the exposed to the unexposed.
- Both designs (**prospective/retrospective**) compare the exposed to the unexposed groups to assess the measure of effect. However, the main distinction between these two designs is calendar time. In the retrospective design, as illustrated in this vignette, exposure to radiation is ascertained from birth data (medical record) and the outcome (thyroid cancer) at the beginning of the study (no follow-up).
- **Cross-sectional** studies, also called surveys and prevalence studies, are designed to assess both the exposure and outcome simultaneously. However, since exposure and disease status

are measured at the same point in time (snapshot), it is difficult, if not impossible, to distinguish whether the exposure preceded or followed the disease, and thus cause-and-effect relationships are not certain, lacking temporal sequence.

- **Ecologic** designs examine group level data in order to establish the relationship between exposure and outcomes.
- A **case-control** design classifies subjects on the basis of outcome (disease and non-disease or comparison group) and then looks backward to identify the exposure. This design could be prospective as well.
  - In this design, the history or previous events for both case and comparison groups are assessed in an attempt to identify the exposure or risk factors for the disease.

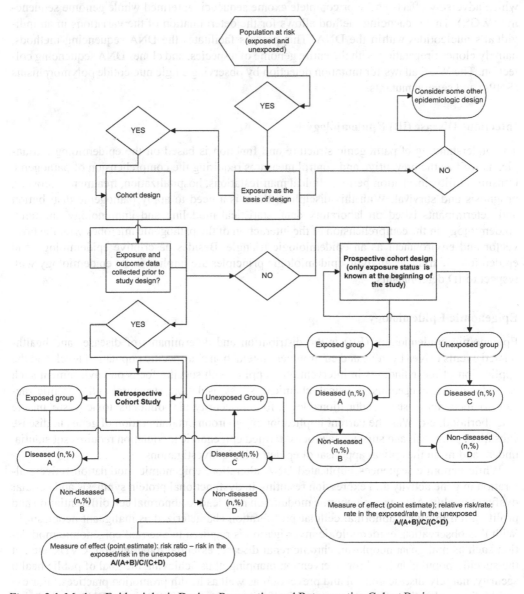

Figure 2.1 Modern Epidemiologic Design: Prospective and Retrospective Cohort Design

Modern Epidemiology and Disease Trajectory

With scientific inquiries utilizing dynamic and not static data in clinical and public health decision making, the notion and concept of epidemiology remains transitional. The early 2000s' human genome project (HGP) facilitated whole genome sequencing (WGS) that provided information on global genomic sequencing in disease causation, implying risk/predisposing factors and etiology. The implication of genomic sequencing in disease processes allow for the reading and interpretation of genetic information in DNA or RNA. For example, the current COVID-19 pandemic allows for genomic sequencing of SARS-CoV2 with respect to mutant strains and variant origin.

The DNA variations outside the exons influence gene expression and protein synthesis, which adversely affects entire or complete exome sequencing, termed whole genome sequencing (WGS). This sequencing method allows for the determination of the variations in an individual's nucleotides within the DNA. This process facilitates the DNA sequencing methods, namely clones preparation with the entire genome of a species, and clones DNA sequencing collection. The WGS allows for mutation detection by observing single nucleotide polymorphisms (SNPs) and several mutants.

Infectious Disease (ID) Epidemiology

The understanding of pathogenic structure and function is based on the epidemiologic triangle, as well as the preventive and control measures requiring the comprehension of pathogenic transmissibility, incubation period, clinical manifestations, hospitalization, treatment, recovery, prognosis and survival. With this discipline, there is a need to apply pathogenic distribution and determinants based on laboratory data, statistical modeling and immunology, immune-epidemiology in the comprehension of the interaction of the pathogenic microbes with the host, vector and environment as an epidemiologic triangle. Besides descriptive epidemiology and epidemiologic triangle, analytic epidemiologic principles are implied in ID epidemiology with respect to ID determinants.

Epigenomic Epidemiology

Epigenomic epidemiology (EE) is the distribution and determinants of disease- and health-related events driven by gene and environment interaction at a specific population level, and the application of these findings in intervention mapping with specific focus on environment such as endogenous, exogenous, physical, chemical, stress, isolation, structural and systemic racism, socioeconomic status, educational level, food insecurity, air pollutants, toxic waste, unsafe neighborhood, etc. With the current implication of environmental alteration of genes in disease causation, prognosis and survival, a process termed epigenomic modulation requires substantial understanding in the critical appraisal of epidemiologic investigations.

While genomic sequences implicated DNA alteration, epigenomic modulation reflects alteration in gene activity and expression resulting in dysfunctional protein synthesis and cellular dysfunctionality. Aberrant epigenomic modulation may lead to abnormal cell differentiation and proliferation implying abnormal cellular proliferation characterized as malignant neoplasm.[2, 3] With this observation, epidemiologic investigation is required in aberrant epigenomic modulation such as malignant neoplasm, chronic renal disease, essential hypertension, CVDs, etc., at the specific population level for intervention mapping, thus achieving the goal of public health security, namely disease control and prevention as well as health promotion practices.[4] For example, the application of whole genome bisulfite sequencing (WGBS) in the DNA methylation

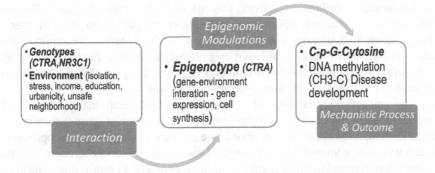

Figure 2.2 Epigenomic Mechanistic Process – DNA Methylation in Epigenomic Epidemiology

Notes: Epigenomic modulation via Methyl group (CH3) – Methyl-cytosine and Transcriptome Inhibition and inverse gene expression ~ Impaired protein synthesis ~ Cellular dysfunctionality and abnormal proliferation.

of the CpG region of the gene allows for the observation of aberrant epigenomic modulation, resulting in specific risk characterization and induction therapy prior to the standard of care. This imitative enhances the role of epidemiology in disease determinants and the application of such data in disease control and optimal preventive services.

Epidemiology today remains translational and epigenomic, implying translational epigenomic epidemiology in meeting the assessment core function of public health as well as individual patient therapeutics. While public health reflects what we as society could do to remain healthy, implying optimal preventive care, clinical medicine requires disease and health intervention. With epidemiology as a basic and applied science in medicine, healthcare providers, mainly physicians, require training in the process of preventing disease recurrence in individual patients. Subsequently, while disease treatment remains the main focus of care in clinical medicine, the healthcare providers' understanding of the environment of individual patients, and the impact of such environment in disease causation, association, etiology, prognosis and mortality, remains a feasible pathway in disease control and prevention at the specific population level.[5]

Epigenomic modulation, which is the gene and environment interaction, primarily involves a methylation process (CH3), which results in DNA methylation as mainly hypermethylation, implying adverse gene expression and downregulation. As stress, isolation and racial/ethnic discrimination impacts social signal transduction, this process results in the binding of CH3 at the non-coding region of the gene termed, the CpG binds to the cytosine leading to methyl cytosine (CH3-G). With the elaboration of CH3-G, there remains impaired transcriptome leading to inverse gene expression, protein synthesis downregulation, marginalized drug receptors, and cellular dysfunctionality as abnormal cellular proliferation.[3,5,6] The US subpopulations with aberrant epigenomic modulations such as racial/ethnic minorities are more predisposed to increase disease incidence, poor prognosis, excess mortality and marginalized survival.

The environmental alteration driven by CO_2 emission, air pollutants and particulates, toxic waste and climate warming adversely affects animals and human-animal biologic systems. Clinical medicine recognized, from its inception, the genetic as well as the environmental predisposition to disease and prognosis. However, if there is a genetic predisposition to a given disease, such manifestations present with higher incidence among families with such defective genes relative to those without such hereditary implication. Additionally, among those with a family history of such conditions, namely essential hypertension (HTN), and stressful environments, such as isolation and subordination at work, this risk of HTN remains higher.[4,5] This observation clearly implicates aberrant genomic modulations in this predisposition, however, in this clinical presentation, such disease progression is not reversible (aberrant genomics) although it is transgenerational. With respect to aberrant epigenomic modulation that reflects the hyper or hypo DNA methylation at the non-coding enhancer region of the gene, this mechanistic process that alters gene expression remains transgenerational although reversible.

Epigenomic epidemiology is the study of distribution and determinants of aberrant epigenomic modulation at the specific population level. The application of these data in specific risk characterization and treatment induction prior to the standard of care, as well as optimal preventive care services, thus addresses the incidence of disease involved in epigenomic modulation as gene expression dysregulation. Epidemiology, in order to assist clinical medicine and public health, must focus on the gene and environment interaction mechanistic process in disease incidence reduction, as well as environmental modification with respect to DNA methylation of the candidate genes in impaired gene expression and marginalized transcriptomes, which adversely affects drug response due to the unavailability of protein molecules as drug receptors. Additionally, given the multifactorial in disease etiology, epidemiology requires the application of translational as well as transdisciplinary trajectories in the assessment of disease determinants for feasible and effective intervention mapping.

Public Health and Epidemiology Integration

Epidemiology remains the foundation of public health. As observed earlier in this chapter, epidemiology is a basic and applied science of clinical medicine and public health, implying its role in the core function of public health, namely assessment of health, disease, injury, disability, natural disaster, pandemics and health-related phenomena at a specific population level. The core function of public health reflects the assessment of the health and health-related phenomena and the application of scientific evidence in data-driven health policy and in assurance, implying essential health services at the community level. In meeting the assessment (A) component of the public health core functions (Assessment (A) Policy (P) Assurance (A)), epidemiology is utilized in addressing the understanding of the disease spectrum as observed in infectious and chronic disease, natural history of disease, subpopulations/community diagnosis and screening, disease risk and predisposing factors, identification of disease precursors, effectiveness of intervention, epidemics, endemics and pandemics investigation for disease control and preventive strategies and the assessment of the effectiveness of public health intentions.[2]

The integrative role of epigenomic epidemiology in public health requires the societal identification of several environments that determine the social gradient, physical, chemical, physiochemical, exogenous and endogenous, in disease etiology. With these specific environments, epigenomic epidemiology enables the understanding of how these environments adversely influence gene expression resulting in gene dysregulation, cellular dysfunctionality and disease development and progression at the specific population level.[4,5] For example, the assessment of DNA methylation of the angiotensin converting enzyme (ACE) gene in a specific population with environmental differentials, such as zip codes, allows for the understanding of aberrant epigenomic modulation at such a geographic locale and intervention mapping involving environmental transformation, induction therapy following specific risk characterization and standard anti-hypertensive therapeutics.

Since environmental conditions, such as social, psychologic, physical, chemical, isolation, social stress, exogenous, endogenous, toxic waste, air pollutions, violent and unsafe neighborhood, social gradient, structural and systemic racism, social injustice and low socioeconomic status, predispose to disease development, prognosis and mortality outcomes, pandemic mitigation and ultimate eradication requires public health initiatives in aberrant epigenomic assessment. With such an approach, future pandemics will transition early to epidemic curve flattening, resulting in pandemic stabilization and marginalization.

Ecologic Non-Experimental Epidemiologic Design

Ecologic designs, also termed group-level ecologic studies, correlational studies, or aggregate studies, obtain data at the level of a group or community often by making use of routinely collected data. Second, if the population, rather than the individual, is the unit of study and its analysis, such a study is correctly characterized as ecologic based on the SARS-CoV2 and COVID-19 data from the local, city and county health departments in the US. This design involves the comparison of aggregate data on risk factors and disease prevalence from different population groups in order to identify associations. Basically, ecologic design or aggregate study refers to an observational study in which all variables are group measures, implying the group as the unit of analysis, in contrast with either a case-control or prospective cohort design where the unit of analysis is the individual level measure. Because all data are aggregated at the group level, relationships at the individual level cannot be empirically determined but are, rather, inferred. Therefore, due to the likelihood of an ecologic fallacy, this design is indicative of weak empirical evidence.

Cross-Sectional Non-Experimental Epidemiologic Design

A cross-sectional design is an observational epidemiologic design that is feasible and ethical when a randomized clinical trial cannot be conducted and other non-experimental designs are less feasible or inefficient. This design basically assesses the association between diseases or health-related events and other variables or factors of interest as potential risk factors in a defined population at a particular time. Contrary to the sampling method involved in case-control design, cross-sectional studies obtain data on exposure and disease status at the same time, implying the prevalence measure and not disease incidence data.

A cross-sectional design is used to measure the prevalence of health outcomes, health determinants, or both in a population at a single point in time or over a short period. Such information can be used to explore disease risk factors. A conducted study to examine demographic and lifestyle predictors of the intention to use a female condom in a defined/specific women population, observed prevalence of the intent to use a female condom was the response or outcome, while demographic and lifestyle variables were the predictors, independent or explanatory variables, and were both measured at the same time from a survey instrument. Since exposure (demographics and lifestyle) and outcome (intent to use a condom) were measured simultaneously for each subject, the cross-sectional nature qualified the design used by these authors. In this study, the authors first identified the population of persons for the study and determined the presence or absence of the intent to use a condom and the lifestyle and demographics for each subject. Using a 2 x 2 table, they compared the prevalence of lifestyle and demographic features in those with the intent to use a female condom and compared it with those without the intent to use female condom: $(A/A+C) \div (B/B+D)$. A cross-sectional design represents a snapshot of the population at a certain point in time.[7]

Because of the inability to establish the cause-and-effect relationship, any association in this design must be interpreted with caution. Second, bias may arise because of selection into or out

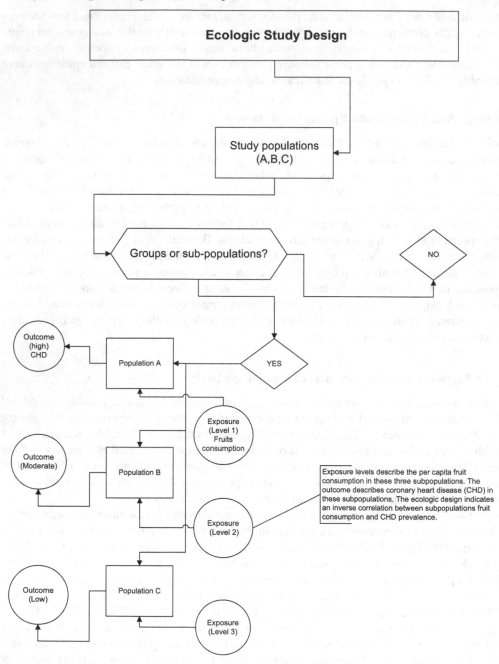

Figure 2.3 Ecologic Design – Non-Individual but Group Data Design

of the study population. Therefore, due to the issues arising from lack of temporality (cause-and-effect relationship), cross-sectional studies of causal association require careful interpretation and recommendation of the findings in control and preventive measures for SARS-CoV2 transmission reduction and COVID-19 mortality marginalization.

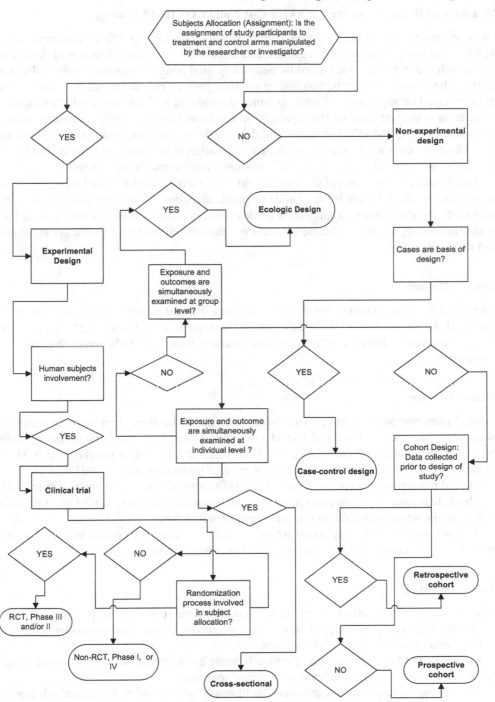

Figure 2.4 Cross-Sectional Non-Experimental Design

Note: This design illustrates the rationale in selection and cross-sectional design as a non-experimental epidemiologic method.

Measures of Disease Occurrence: SARS-CoV2 and COVID-19 Analogy

There are many steps in the epidemiologic investigation of this COVID-19 pandemic, one of which is the association between exposure and disease development. Measures of disease association include, but are not limited to, commonly used point estimates in epidemiologic research. These measures can be absolute or relative, such as risk difference and relative risk, respectively. The application of such measures depends on multiple steps, which involve an association in the first place and the establishment of factual association by eliminating random error, confounding and effect measure modifiers, as the possible explanation of such association. The commonly used measures of disease association or nexus include, but are not limited to, relative odds or odds ratio, relative risk, risk ratio, coefficient and hazard ratio.

Additionally, the measures of disease comparison are interchangeably used with measures of association or effect. Below is the formula to enable clinicians, biomedical researchers, public health officers and students to apply these crude measures of effect in understanding these basic epidemiologic approaches to disease association, relationship and effect. Below are the simplified approaches.

Absolute Measure

Subtracted from one another and provide information about public health impact of an exposure. If the prevalence of SARS-CoV2 is 21.5% in population A, and 31.5% in population B, the prevalence difference reflects absolute measure, which is 10.0% comparing these two populations.

Relative Measure

Divided from one another, and provide information about the strength of the relationship between exposure (independent variable) and outcome (disease, disabilities, or injuries). If the risk in population A based on SARS-CoV2 infection is 21.5 and the risk in population B is 31.5%, the relative risk is determined by the risk in the exposed population (B), divided by the risk in the unexposed population A, implying Exposed (31.5)/Unexposed (21.5), with the risk ratio >1.00.

Absolute measures of comparison are risk difference, rate difference, incidence rate difference, cumulative incidence difference, and prevalence difference.

Relative measures of comparison are risk ratio, rate ratio, relative rate or relative risk, incidence rate ratio, cumulative incidence ratio, and prevalence ratio.

Rate versus Risk

Risk is the accumulated effect of rate occurring during some specified time period.

Risk has no time dimension, and the reference population in risk is the population unaffected at the beginning of the period of observation.

Attack Rate (AR), although not specifically a rate but a proportion, is the cumulative incidence of a disease during an outbreak or transient epidemic.

AR = Diseased (exposed and developed an illness)/Diseased and Non-diseased (all exposed to the suspected agent of contamination) x (multiplier [100]) during a time period.

Secondary Attack Rate (SAR) is the proportion of individuals exposed to the primary case (primary cases), who themselves develop the disease (secondary cases).

SAR = Number of new cases in group minus initial case(s)/Number of susceptible persons in a group − Initial case(s).

Table 2.1 Measures of Comparison/Association/Relationship/Nexus/Correlation

Measure	Formula	Explanation
Rate or Risk Ratio (RR)	*RE/RU*, where *RE* = risk or rate in the exposed and *RU* = risk or rate in the unexposed	Measures the strength of association between exposure and the disease (outcome)
Attributable proportion among total population	*(RT − RU) / RT* x **100**, where *RT* = incidence rate (IR), cumulative incidence (CI), or prevalence proportion (PP) in the total population and *RU* is the IR, CI, or PP in the unexposed population	Measures the excess proportion of disease in the total population, assuming the exposure is causal and implying that the proportion of a disease in a total population that would be eliminated if the exposure were eliminated
Attributable proportion among the exposed	*(RE − RU) / RE* x **100**	Measures the proportion of disease among the exposed, assuming the exposure is causal and implying the proportion of disease among the exposed that will be eliminated if the exposure is eliminated
Population rate difference	*RT − RU* or *RD* x *PE*, where *RD* = IR difference, CI difference, or PP difference; and *PE* = proportion of population that is exposed, and *RD* = *RE − RU*	Measures excess rate or risk of a disease or outcome in the total population
Rate or Rate Difference	RE − RU	Measures rate or risk of disease or outcome among the exposed population
Attack rate	*ND/TP*, where *ND* = number of people at risk in whom a certain outcome develops, and *TP* = total number of people at risk	Compares the risk of outcome in groups with different exposure

Notes and Abbreviations: RE = Rate parameter such as risk among the exposed; RU = Rate parameter or point estimate among the unexposed.

Epidemiologic Data Interpretation

Epidemiologic objectives remain the identification of populations at risk and the application of such knowledge to disease prevention and control. Clinical medicine is comparable given that the clinicians addressing COVID-19 patients have an obligation to prevent death in the process of treating disease and prevent complications following treatment, thus maintaining health. Within this context, epidemiologic principles and methods are applied by clinicians in the process of minimizing therapeutic complications, prolonging survival, and maintaining the health of COVID-19 patients.

The objective of clinical research is to provide valid and reliable evidence regarding therapeutics, screening, diagnostics, and prevention and depends on the design as well as the statistical methods used to generate these results. Clinical research designs are broadly classified as non-experimental and experimental or clinical trials if conducted in human populations. This (clinical) evidence is presented as measures of the effects of disease, treatment, procedure or screening, etc. These effects are described as absolute or relative measures of comparison. Absolute measures of comparison describe and quantify the differences between two measures of disease frequency, while relative measures of comparison describe and quantify ratios of two measures of frequency, as well as the strength of association or relationship between exposure and the outcome of interest. For example, the rate difference measures the excess rate of outcome or disease among the exposed patient population, while relative rate compares the rate in the exposed with the unexposed and indicates the strength of the relationship between the exposed and the disease or outcome. The rates of disease or outcome obtained from clinical studies may be compared across different study populations, but the reliability of such comparisons require adjusted rates (for example, age-adjusted rate), also termed standardized rates.

Understanding the interpretation of these measures is essential to the application of the findings in clinical research to the improvement of patient care as well as population health. Therefore, although sound statistical methods and inference are highly relevant in clinical studies, it is very important to apply accurate epidemiologic methods or the principles of the design of an investigation, since valid evidence cannot be obtained unless the design is sound and accurate. Finally, because clinical research or epidemiologic studies are often entangled with confounding, caution is required in the interpretation of measures of disease occurrence or effects where these factors are not adjusted and illustrated in the crude or raw measures of association.

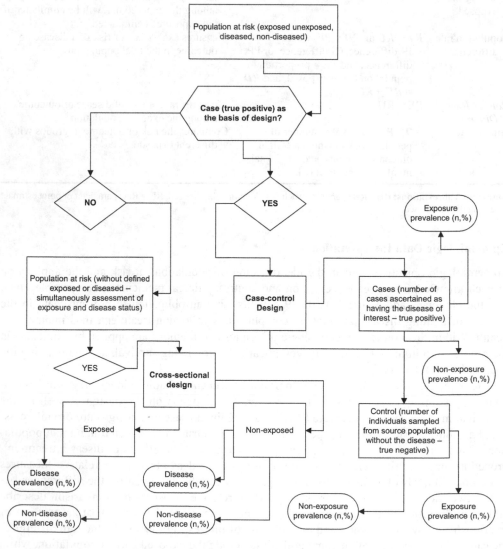

Figure 2.5 Cross-Sectional Study Design versus Case-Control Study Design

Questions for Discussion

1. Describe the role of immuno-epidemiology in SARS-CoV2 and COVID-19 control and prevention.
2. Explain: (a) ecologic epidemiologic design in SARS-CoV2 case-fatality and mortality assessment and (b) cross-sectional non-experimental design in COVID-19 mortality assessment at subpopulation level.
3. Describe the measures of association in epidemiologic design.
4. With respect to descriptive epidemiology, describe SARS-CoV2 with respect to host, agent and environment.
5. With respect to SARS-CoV2 and COVID-19, how could you explain the epigenomic epidemiology perspective in the assessment of the environment and the application of such data in prevention and control?
6. Explain epidemiology and public health integration in viral pandemic mitigation, marginalization and the return to pre-pandemic era.

Notes

1 "Epidemiology: The Foundation of Public Health". http://www.ph.ucla.edu/epi/faculty/detels/PH150/ Detels_Epidemiology.pdf. Accessed 9 Mar. 2022.
2 Holmes L, Jr, Opara, F. *Concise Epidemiologic Principles and Concepts: Guidelines for Clinicians and Biomedical Researchers*. Author House, 2013.
3 Holmes, L Jr, Lim A, Okundaye, O. et al. DNA Methylation of Candidate Genes (ACE II, IFN-γ, AGTR 1, CKG, ADD1, SCNN1B and TLR2) in Essential Hypertension: A Systematic Review and Quantitative Evidence Synthesis. *Int J Environ Res Public Health*, 2019; 16(23): 4829. doi: 10.3390/ ijerph16234829.
4 Holmes L Jr, Shutman E, Chinaka C, Deepika K, Pelaez L, Dabney KW. Aberrant Epigenomic Modulation of Glucocorticoid Receptor Gene (NR3C1) in Early Life Stress and Major Depressive Disorder Correlation: Systematic Review and Quantitative Evidence Synthesis. *Int J Environ Res Public Health*, 4 November 2019; 16(21): 4280. doi: 10.3390/ijerph16214280.
5 Holmes L, Chinaka C, Elmi H, Deepika K, Pelaez L, Enwere M, Akinola OT, Dabney KW. Implication of Spiritual Network Support System in Epigenomic Modulation and Health Trajectory. *Int J Environ Res Public Health*, 25 October 2019; 16(21): 4123. doi: 10.3390/ijerph16214123.
6 Holmes, L Jr, Ogungbade, GO, Ward, DD, et al. Potential Markers of Female Condom Use among Inner City African-American Women. *AIDS Care*, 2008; 20(4): 470–477. doi: 10.1080/09540120701867016.
7 Holmes, L. Jr. *Applied Epidemiologic Principles and Concepts: Clinicians' Guide to Study Design and Conduct*. Taylor & Francis, 2018.

3 SARS-CoV2 (COVID-19)

Pandemic and Public Health Emergency Response

Scientific Reality in Disease Modeling and Epidemic Curve Plateau/Flattening

While epidemiology reflects disease distribution and determinants at a specific population level, the understanding of the exponential SARS-CoV2 spread process and trajectory enables viral pathogenic spread marginalization. Additionally, the application of the observed data on pathogenic spread facilitates the pathway in curve flattening in pandemics. The application of data on the pathogenic tracing, tracking and testing as "3Ts" during the pandemic enables stabilization and marginalization of pathogenic transmission, and mutants or variants.

Epidemiologic Transition and Curve

Epidemiologic data reflect a transition from infectious disease as the leading cause of death in the 1900s to chronic disease namely CVDs in the current era. This scientific experience provided a substantial amount of data to epidemiology on infectious disease modeling in terms of transmission, incubation period, subclinical disease, infectivity, prognosis and fatality.[1] Additionally, epidemiologic approaches to infectious disease observed epidemic curves which could be due to excess fatality or transmission containment and mitigation through intense screening and pathogen detection.

Current Global Pandemic

The coronavirus, characterized as SARS-CoV2, a causative pathogen in COVID-19, meaning a special antigenic type of coronavirus disease causing pathogen discovered in 2019, remains a pandemic. This microbe is an intracellular pathogen, meaning that it requires the host cells of humans in order to replicate and continue to survive! Genetically, this is a single stranded enveloped RNA virus with a specialized means of gene expression for its genomic stability and proliferation.[2] Unlike its previous antigenic type or variants, the SARS-CoV2 RNA transcriptome is very pathogenic and highly virulent, meaning an extremely contagious and disease-causing pathogenic microbe.

SARS-CoV2 Transmission

The SARS-CoV2 microbe is transmitted from person-to-person as a community-acquired pathogen. The mode of transmission includes viral droplets from the nose, eyes and mouth, with the droplet able to survive on several surfaces for over 24 hours. Individuals who are infected with this microbe may transmit the virus to others, even though such individuals do not manifest any symptoms, they are termed carriers and are asymptomatic.[3]

DOI: 10.4324/9781003424451-3

Manifestations/Symptoms

The manifestations of COVID-19 include dry and productive cough, fever, sneezing, shortness of breath, tiredness as decreased vitality, and lower respiratory tract colonization including pneumonia. While fever is a protective mechanism for the host in order to limit pathogen replication, it may result in extracellular fluid imbalance, requiring fluid consumption during any viral pandemic. However, individuals can be infected with this virus without fever, especially if such individuals are immuno-incompetent, implying compromised immune system response. The history of infectious disease is very clear, as it is not clinically beneficial to treat the fever of an infection with an antipyretic agent, however, fever could be regulated to avoid seizure, especially in children, by low/moderate application of antipyretics.[4] Again, the role of fever in an infection is to provide protection to the host by limiting viral replication via pathogenic transcriptome denaturation. The excessive use of ibuprofen, for example, in the context of a novel pathogen within the community without antibodies to the pathogen, is indicative of excessive viral replication and the inability of human interferon gamma to protect the non-infected human cells against the virally infected cells, and the subsequent cellular dysfunction and extreme community fatality. This leads, in part, to the explanation of the fever dysregulation in coronavirus fatality! Specifically, when the immune system is compromised, there remains an increased risk of infection and mortality, requiring the immune system potentiation in epidemic curve flattening!

Population at Risk and Subpopulations Transmissibility and Fatality Disparities

With most microbes, there is an increased risk of infection in the elderly because of the decline in biologic function including their immune system such as antibody response to a given antigen or epitope, children with chronic diseases such as moderate or severe asthma, the chronically ill with COPD, asthma, Type 2 diabetes, cancer patients on chemotherapy, drug and substance users/abusers,[5] alcoholics with impaired immune system response, etc. With the limited resources of the healthcare system with respect to test kits, negative pressure rooms, ventilators, personal protective equipment, decontaminants, and quarantine space, racial/ethnic minorities except Asian Americans in the US, characterized with public insurance (Medicare and Medicaid), underserved, and poor (low socioeconomic status) and those residing in disadvantaged social neighborhoods with increased psychosocial stress remain disproportionately affected by SARS-CoV2 (6).[6] SARS-CoV2 control and prevention should apply equitable resources in the curve flattening, since failure to do so by any healthcare system or public health institution in the world will lead to a kurtosis or peak in the epidemic curve.

Diagnosis/Detection/Treatment

Diagnosis involves the use of high-throughput RNA sequencing to detect the viral antigen in terms of the transcriptome, the specific RNA as a polymeric molecule and not antibody detection. The management of COVID-19 involves the treatment of symptoms in the upper and lower respiratory tract involving ABC, meaning airway,[7] breathing and circulation via ventilators, and other symptoms management. Currently, there is no antiviral agent for SARS-CoV2 (COVID-19), while a vaccine for antibody production is anticipated months from now, if not a couple of years.

Prevention and Control of Transmission

The primary measures of COVID-19 control and prevention require the utilization of rigorous hand washing once individuals have been in contact with unknown and unfamiliar surfaces, personal protective equipment for healthcare workers and infectious disease epidemiologists, avoidance of hugging and kissing as well as restricted facial touching mainly the mouth, eyes and nose. In addition, to limit the spread, we recommend avoiding crowds and large gatherings such as in churches, Muslim places of worship, Hindu temples and Jewish places of worship, movies and restaurants, and apply hand sanitizer during grocery shopping and at gas/diesel pumps. Also, because this microbe is not transmitted by air droplets but by contact, the use of a mask remains very useful in controlling its spread, as well as feasible in healthcare settings, as personal protective equipment, in mitigating nosocomial infections. Further, "closed cohort" such as nursing homes and prisons should restrict visitations.[8] There is a need to increase the screening of individuals suspected of upper and lower respiratory tract infections and require local, county, state and federal Public Health Departments to accelerate the screening processes and adhere to infectious disease control protocol, if epidemic curve flattening is feasible and hence reduce transmission and fatality from this highly contagious microbe. Since fatality prevalence and not rate depends on immunopotentiation, resources are required for those with low SES in enhancing balanced nutrients during this period, thus increasing immune response.[9] Furthermore, by restricting travel, except for essential services, SARS-CoV2 spread remains marginalized.

Epidemic Curve Flattening

The intense screening of suspected cases, healthcare workers and residents in nursing homes and prisons, and the restricted use of public transportation such as buses and trains, except for necessary travel, could assist in curve flattening. Further, as we recommend the potentiation of the immune system via innate (neutrophil and macrophage elaboration) and acquired or specific (immunoglobulins and CD4 cells) immune response to antigen or pathogen, SARS-CoV2 transmission could be reduced with respect to fatality proportion or prevalence, hence epidemic curve flattening.[10] Should the global epidemic require flattening by May 2020, these suggestions for global public health response must be implemented. Consequently, since all scientific data involves some element of uncertainty, and hence the application of p values in the quantification of random error, the predictive modeling on coronavirus, SARS-CoV2 and COVID-19 curve flattening by May 2020 may be negatively influenced by a global lack of case detection resources, as well as the non-adherence to infectious disease control and prevention protocols.

Questions for Discussion

1. What is a viral pandemic and how could this concept be applied to the epidemiologic triangle?
2. Describe epidemic curve and explain the factors resulting in epidemiologic curve flattening.
3. Suppose there is a future viral pandemic, what are the epidemiologic directives in viral tracing, tracking and testing?
4. Briefly discuss the role of public health emergency response in viral pathogenic transmission marginalization.

Notes

1 "The Epidemiologic Transition: Changing Patterns of Mortality and …". https://www.ncbi.nlm.nih.gov/pmc/articles/PMC2805833/. Accessed 12 Nov. 2021.
2 "Virology in the 21st Century – NCBI". 18 Mar. 2009, https://www.ncbi.nlm.nih.gov/pmc/articles/PMC2681991/. Accessed 12 Nov. 2021.

3 "Transmission of SARS-CoV-2: Implications for Infection Prevention". 9 Jul. 2020, https://www.who.int/news-room/commentaries/detail/transmission-of-sars-cov-2-implications-for-infection-prevention-precautions. Accessed 12 Nov. 2021.

4 "COVID-19 Basics N Harvard Health". https://www.health.harvard.edu/diseases-and-conditions/covid-19-basics. Accessed 12 Nov. 2021.

5 "Aging, Immunity, and COVID-19: How Age Influences the Host ...". 12 Jan. 2021, https://www.frontiersin.org/articles/10.3389/fphys.2020.571416/full. Accessed 12 Nov. 2021.

6 "PCD: US Public Health Response to COVID-19 and Chronic Disease". 1 Aug. 2020, https://www.cdc.gov/pcd/collections/pdf/US-Public-Health-Response-to-COVID-19.pdf. Accessed 12 Nov. 2021.

7 RNA as a Stable Polymer to Build Controllable and Defined ... – NCBI". https://www.ncbi.nlm.nih.gov/pmc/articles/PMC4707685/. Accessed 12 Nov. 2021

8 "Factors Involved in the Aerosol Transmission of Infection and Control ...". https://www.ncbi.nlm.nih.gov/pmc/articles/PMC7114857/. Accessed 12 Nov. 2021.

9 "Community Mitigation Framework | CDC". https://www.cdc.gov/coronavirus/2019-ncov/community/community-mitigation.html. Accessed 12 Nov. 2021.

10 "Prevention and Control of COVID-19 in Nursing Homes, Orphanages ...". 2 Jul. 2020, https://www.ncbi.nlm.nih.gov/pmc/articles/PMC7332257/. Accessed 12 Nov. 2021.

4   SARS-CoV2 Mutation
Immuno-Epidemiologic and Socio-Epidemiologic response

SARS-CoV2 Mutations/Strains

The mutation or alteration of a viral or bacterial microbe reflects the epitope or antigenic variance with time and exposure, implying antigenic subtypes and variants of such microbe. Specifically, or simply, the less mutated a pathogen or microbe is, the more stable its epitopes (antigen presenting sites of a microbe) and antigenicity, indicative of an improved immune response with stable antibody production and subsequent immune complex generation, thus enhancing immuno-potentiation and self-protection.[1] The pandemic nature of this microbe and its mutation stability is indicative of the stable although aberrant epigenomic modulation of COVID-19. With SARS-CoV2 observed to be stable in terms of mutation, vaccine availability will enhance reliable antibody production, improve prognosis and decrease fatality.[2]

SARS-CoV2 Mutation Implication in Clinical Manifestations and Severity

In addressing COVID-19 fatality, should this pathogen continue and reappear after this pandemic, humanity, regardless of age, class, sex, religious beliefs and other socio-demographics, should be immunized against SARS-CoV2. Additionally, since antibody availability in terms of immuno-potentiation depends on glycoprotein,[3] enhancing antibodies to COVID-19, humans as hosts require healthy and balanced nutrition including more fruit and vegetable consumption in dietary plans and schedules. The current immuno-epidemiological response to SARS-CoV2 mutation signals optimism in therapeutic and prophylactic approaches to COVID-19 reinfection and future episodes.[4] The observed stable mutation of SARS-CoV2 is suggestive of improved prognosis following a reinfection from COVID-19 during this pandemic, which is possible as the pandemic continues globally.

In summary, viral pathogenic with less mutation or novel strains remains a pathway to epidemic curve flattening as well as community herd immunity optimization and population spread reduction. With several antigenic subtypes as variants or mutants, the more challenging are the vaccination initiatives and the need to address population densities. Since viral pathogens require mutations for survivability based on human host ability to downregulate their survival via antibodies, T-cell and NK-cell integration, the lesser the SARS-CoV2 variants or mutants, the more likely the epidemic curve flattening if social and physical distancing, face mask wearing and rigorous hand washing are considered as appropriate measures for control and prevention.

Socio-Epidemiologic Response

Descriptive epidemiology requires the knowledge of place, person and time that allows for the application of dynamic data in disease control, mitigation and prevention. With such initiatives,

DOI: 10.4324/9781003424451-4

the scientific community and public health evolves the epidemiologic triangle, namely, host (humans), agent (SARS-CoV2) and environment (social, psychosocial, psychological, isolation, physical, chemical, etc.) in pathogenic microbe mitigation and risk reduction. This chapter observes the geographic variances that implicate several risk factors in SARS-CoV2 transmissibility and spread, as well as the potential response in spread stabilization and mitigation.

Social Risk Factors in COVID-19 Pandemic

Epidemiology reflects distribution and predisposing factors as well as risk determinants in a given disease and health-related events (pregnancy, natural disaster). With an epidemiologic triangle with respect to pathogenic spread in a specific human population, there is a need to examine: (a) humans as host, (b) SARS-CoV2 as the agent and (c) environment such as physical, psychological, social, psychosocial, economic, toxic waste, isolation, discrimination, health insurance coverage, etc. The social epidemiologic response to SARS-CoV2 transmission implies community effort via the healthcare system at the local, county, state and national levels in applying scientific and reliable approaches to testing, tracing and tracking of individuals with seropositivity in order to address the epidemiologic curve flattening, spread stabilization and marginalization.

COVID-19 Case Fatalities: Global Health Data

The epidemic and endemic data on COVID-19 indicates Italy (estimated 5.3% fatality proportion) as the global epicenter, followed by Spain (estimated 4.9%). France, rather than China, assuming the data is reliable, already has epidemic curve flattening (no domestic incident COVID-19 cases) as per March 20, 2020. Europe needs to simulate epidemiologic disease modeling, especially distancing, case tracing, and immune system potentiation through innate and acquired or specific response.[5]

Socio-Economic Status (SES) and COVID-19 Fatalities Disparities

With the limited and restricted pathogenic microbes' knowledge of infectivity and immune system potentiation, social and physical distancing protects human lives, implying SARS-CoV2 control measures. As an epidemiologic response to epidemic curve flattening, humans, as SARS-CoV2 hosts, require distancing, an analogy of the human/social laboratory in pandemic mitigation. Despite the consistent effort in encouraging social network support systems, implying interpersonal connectome for gene expression and normal epigenomic modulation, socio-economic enhancement facilitates appropriate and reliable measures in control and prevention of SARS-CoV2 transmission, good prognosis and marginalized mortality. However, specific populations must encourage employability, implying working remotely, given the asymptomatic transmission of SARS-CoV2, a causative pathogen in COVID-19 viral disease.[6] With this directive, pathogenic spread remains marginalized and stabilized.

SARS-CoV2 Transmissibility and Societal Response, US

The societal failure to meet this social epidemiologic response, namely consistent employability, immune system potentiation through stress reduction and appropriate nutrients, case tracing, community COVID-19 education and enhanced screening and testing, increase economic anxiety and strain, as well as "corona-phobia virus" especially among the most vulnerable populations, namely Blacks, Hispanics, American Indians/Alaska Natives[7] and underserved Whites in the US, impairing COVID-19 prognosis among cases and increased mortality and fatality prevalence both nationally and globally.

The current fatality proportion, as per March 20, 2020, in the US was 1.5%, relatively lower than the global fatality proportion of 4.2%. Therefore, it is incredibly important that the US, a nation with health disparities, adheres to social determinants of health (SDH) and social epidemiologic response (SER) in flattening this curve before long, thus lowering the transmission and decreasing the spread of COVID-19 both nationally and globally. Since public health issues in one geographic locale implies a public health crisis everywhere, as human society reflects a global village, ensuring an adequate social epidemiologic response (SER) through social/health equity, implies optimal COVID-19 curve flattening in the US.[8]

Social epidemiologic implication in any viral pandemic requires the understanding of the social determinants of pathogenic risk with respect to transmissibility, treatment, prognosis and mortality outcomes. The descriptive epidemiologic approach in addressing SARS-CoV2 curve flattening, stabilization and marginalization in any community setting, requires the understanding and application of reliable, accurate viral disease control and prevention measures. Since SARS-CoV2 behavior reflects *"catch me if you can"*, SER requires community appropriate testing, tracing and tracking. Further, the application of appropriate and reliable face mask wearing, physical and social distancing and hand washing remain effective measures in the reducing the national and global spread of SARS-CoV2.

Questions for Discussion

1. What role does social factor play in viral pathogenic transmission?
2. Explain the social determinants of health and its role in SARS-CoV2 transmission and infectivity.
3. What is the impact of low SES in SARS-CoV2 subpopulations differentials in transmission and COVID-19 mortality?
4. Describe a viral structure especially SARS-CoV2. Is this pathogen DNA or RNA virus?
5. Explain the notion of the SARS-CoV2 as a non-living organism.
6. Describe viral mutation or strain. Is there any observed mutation in SARS-CoV2?

Notes

1 "Common Strategies for Antigenic Variation by Bacterial, Fungal and …". https://www.ncbi.nlm.nih.gov/pmc/articles/PMC3676878/. Accessed 12 Nov. 2021.
2 The British Variant of the New Coronavirus-19 (Sars-Cov-2 … – PubMed". https://pubmed.ncbi.nlm.nih.gov/33377359/. Accessed 12 Nov. 2021.
3 "Reduced Risk of Reinfection with SARS-CoV-2 After COVID-19 …". 13 Aug. 2021, https://www.cdc.gov/mmwr/volumes/70/wr/mm7032e1.htm. Accessed 12 Nov. 2021.
4 Nutrition and Immunity: Lessons for COVID-19 – NCBI". 23 Jun. 2021, https://www.ncbi.nlm.nih.gov/pmc/articles/PMC8223524/. Accessed 12 Nov. 2021.
5 "How to Flatten the Curve on Coronavirus – The New York Times". 27 Mar. 2020, https://www.nytimes.com/article/flatten-curve-coronavirus.html. Accessed 12 Nov. 2021.
6 "Flattening the Curve for COVID-19: What Does It Mean and How …". 11 Mar. 2020, https://healthblog.uofmhealth.org/wellness-prevention/flattening-curve-for-covid-19-what-does-it-mean-and-how-can-you-help. Accessed 12 Nov. 2021.
7 "Let's Flatten the Infodemic Curve – WHO | World Health Organization". https://www.who.int/newsroom/spotlight/let-s-flatten-the-infodemic-curve. Accessed 12 Nov. 2021.
8 "'Flattening the Curve' May Be the World's Best Bet to Slow … – Stat News". 11 Mar. 2020, https://www.statnews.com/2020/03/11/flattening-curve-coronavirus/. Accessed 12 Nov. 2021.

5 COVID-19 Pandemic

Epidemic Curve Down-Drifting and Case Fatality Mitigation

US and Global Case Fatality Geographic Locale Variance

SARS-CoV2 transmission and case fatality continues to rise daily in the US, with sustained impact in the following states, New York, Michigan, Wisconsin. Illinois, Louisiana, Florida and Massachusetts. COVID-19 curve flattening and case fatality mitigation in the US requires national epidemic curve flattening and case fatality models. These models should be based on reliable epidemiologic data and experience in data projection, forecasting and simulation. We developed an epidemic curve flattening and case fatality model based on COVID-19 testing and case confirmation and mortality in South Korea (SK) and Italy.[1] This model utilized the population size of SK, the number of individuals tested and confirmed cases per day from the onset of testing and case detection and the US Census, 2020, projected population size for simulation.[2]

The US confirmed cases ($n = 277,522$), exceeds any other nation in the world accounting for 24.46% of globally confirmed cases, and case fatality of 2.71%, reflecting an 11.67% of globally confirmed current mortality (April 4, 2020). Germany represents a nation with a very low case fatality ($n = 1.39\%$) despite an increased number of confirmed cases, $n = 91,159$ (8.15%). The number of confirmed cases in SK is 10,156, representing 0.91% of the total global cases ($n = 1,118,304$), with a case fatality of 1.74% ($n = 177$), accounting for 0.30% of worldwide total mortality.[3] With the US confirmed cases' increasing pattern, we anticipate curve flattening with the case fatality at 4.22% if the SK approach to epidemic curve flattening and case fatality mitigation is robustly applied in the US.[4]

US Epidemiologic Curve Flattening

What is curve flattening? This epidemiologic concept reflects the notion of pathogenic microbe transmission control, resulting in less transmission that signals case positivity reduction. This involves the application of transmission down drifting in achieving curve flattening and plateau. In flattening and down drifting the epidemic curve, the US is required to apply the SK case detection and contact tracing initiative strategies that involved: (a) the application of infectious disease diagnostic clinical guidelines by requesting anyone with respiratory tract symptoms and signs to be tested. (b) Anyone who perceives or thinks of being exposed to a case or circumstance that may implicate COVID-19 spread to be tested. (c) Instant contact tracing, tracking and testing of suspected cases. (d) Rapid test and results for isolation, quarantining and hospitalization. (e) Instant isolation and hospitalization/admission for symptoms management, especially intubation and ventilation for ABC improvement.

DOI: 10.4324/9781003424451-5

US Epidemiologic Curve Flattening: Social and Physical Distancing

The mandatory requirement of physical and social distancing is required in all states and US territories. The recommendation of face mask (non-surgical or medical mask) wearing in the community remains mandatory, since asymptomatic individuals or carriers of COVID-19 could transmit the pathogen to unexposed individuals in several communities, accelerating transmission and viral spread.[5] There is a need in all pandemics to apply reliable face masking in pathogenic spread mitigation, thus enhancing community herd immunity.

US Epidemiologic Curve Flattening: Health Inequity and Social Resources Allocation

Health equity reflects the just and fair allocation of social, economic and environmental conditions pertaining to health to all subjects in human society. In a specific population or nation, states, counties, cities and healthcare systems, as well as public health departments, must practice equitable sharing and allocation of resources such as personal protective equipment (PPE), ventilators and healthcare workers for the current pandemic epicenter and peri-epicenter such as New York, Louisiana, Washington, Massachusetts, Illinois and California. The lack of resources and scientific data in pandemics increase case fatalities as well as transmission, given limited PPE in most states, counties and cities' healthcare systems.[6] The unwillingness of states with a few confirmed cases and Americans within the 75th percentile of wealth to allocate resources to these epicenters, may result in the transformation of states with few confirmed cases today to epicenters tomorrow, implying adverse emotional and physical health outcomes for all Americans regardless of social status. In addition, scientists, epidemiologists, infectious disease specialists and researchers should advocate the application of scientific data in flattening the epidemic curve, while anticipating curve down drifting and subsequent case fatality mitigation.[7]

Further, in ensuring COVID-19 spread stabilization and case fatality mitigation, resources should be provided by all socioeconomically advantaged individuals to the socially disadvantaged by ensuring that all Americans regardless of social gradient, are equipped with face masks and other COVID-19 protective equipment.[8] Therefore the collective application of recommended strategies and equitable resource sharing and donation could result in model advantage by flattening the curve sooner than expected in these models, thus reducing and mitigating case fatalities in the US to <100,000 as assumed by the current model utilized by the National COVID-19 Taskforce.

Questions for Discussion

1. Describe epidemic curve in viral pandemic.
2. What is curve flattening and down-drifting?
3. Explain the factors utilized in epidemic curve flattening.
4. Describe the implication of available social resources in epidemic curve flattening and mitigation in several subpopulations.

Notes

1 "Dynamic Panel Surveillance of COVID-19 Transmission – NCBI". https://www.ncbi.nlm.nih.gov/pmc/articles/PMC7546733/. Accessed 12 Nov. 2021.
2 Population Projections – Census Bureau". https://www.census.gov/programs-surveys/popproj.html. Accessed 12 Nov. 2021.

3 "COVID-19 Trends from Germany Show Different Impacts by Gender …". 1 May. 2020, https://www.brookings.edu/blog/techtank/2020/05/01/covid-19-trends-from-germany-show-different-impacts-by-gender-and-age/. Accessed 12 Nov. 2021.

4 "Flattening-the-Curve Associated with Reduced COVID-19 Case Fatality …". 17 Apr. 2020, https://www.ncbi.nlm.nih.gov/pmc/articles/PMC7162747/. Accessed 12 Nov. 2021.

5 COVID-19: Considerations for Wearing Masks | CDC". https://www.cdc.gov/coronavirus/2019-ncov/prevent-getting-sick/cloth-face-cover-guidance.html. Accessed 12 Nov. 2021.

6 "Strategies for Optimizing the Supply of Facemasks: COVID-19 | CDC". https://www.cdc.gov/coronavirus/2019-ncov/hcp/ppe-strategy/face-masks.html. Accessed 12 Nov. 2021.

7 "Flattening the Curve is Flattening the Complexity of Covid-19 – NCBI". 10 Feb. 2021, https://www.ncbi.nlm.nih.gov/pmc/articles/PMC7874568/. Accessed 12 Nov. 2021.

8 "Contributing Factors to Personal Protective Equipment Shortages – NCBI". 2 Oct. 2020, https://www.ncbi.nlm.nih.gov/pmc/articles/PMC7531934/. Accessed 12 Nov. 2021.

6 Pregnancy Risk in SARS-CoV2 Transmission and COVID-19 Fetal Survivability

Immuno-Epidemiologic Perspective

Human Immune System Interaction in Pregnancy (Fetal Development)

The immune system cascade remains altered during pregnancy due to the fetal cells conveying paternal antigens that might provoke gestational/maternal immune response, inducing miscarriage or preterm birth. Simply, the fundamental role of the human immune system is to protect the host "self" against "non-self" or antigen as illustrated by the innate and specific immune response to a presenting pathogen or antigen.[1] If the oocytes or fetal cells are perceived by the maternal immune system as "foreign", antigen or non-self, there is a tendency for the rejection of the embryo at the uterine implantation site, resulting in miscarriage. Also, maternal immune systems may be associated, in part, with preterm birth.[2]

Whereas the analogy of organ transplant might reflect embryonic uterine implantation, it is not an accurate characterization of gestational immunogenicity, due to the maternal immune system modulation between pro-inflammatory and anti-inflammatory response during the trimesters of pregnancy.[3] While it is no longer accurate to claim immune system repression during pregnancy, it is scientifically accurate to support the pregnancy alteration of the normal immune response with respect to non-adaptive or innate and adaptive or specific immune response. Whereas the regulatory T cells are important in immuno-potentiation during pregnancy, on average viral pathogens have the tendency to deactivate the immune system, resulting in impaired response of interferon -γ in protecting the non-virally infected cells against viral replication.[4] Since the maternal immune system is in alteration mode due to this influx, there is an increased risk of immuno-compromisation with COVID-19, predisposing pregnancy to increased risk of transmission and infectivity. In addition, the interaction between the fetal cells and maternal immune system may result in fetal infection by COVID-19.[5]

The recommendation of breastfeeding if the mother is infected and recovered from symptoms but still positive for COVID-19 should not be considered in this pandemic. While breast milk contains an estimated 75–80% of secretory immunoglobulin (SIgA), 10–15% of IgM and IgG and natural killer cells (NKCs) which have been shown to be protective against respiratory infection,[6] gastrointestinal disorders and neurodegeneration, its recommendation must weigh between the risk and benefit, despite the claim of SARS-CoV2 absence in breast milk based on limited data.

Spontaneous Abortion Risk Reduction and Vaccine Uptake

With the observed spontaneous abortion in viral pandemics, vaccine recommendation remains vital. The current immuno-epidemiologic perspective suggests:

1. Testing of all pregnant/expecting mothers with respiratory manifestations with respect to SARS-CoV2 seropositivity.

DOI: 10.4324/9781003424451-6

2. Identification and testing of all expectant mothers in contact with suspected or confirmed COVID-19 cases as well as all pregnant mothers who wish to, or express interest in testing.[7]
3. Contact tracing and testing of all individuals exposed to or in contact with confirmed COVID-19 expected mothers.
4. Social and physical distancing for all pregnant/expecting mothers.
5. Isolation, admission and hospitalization of all confirmed pregnant cases.
6. Application of face masks, especially among pregnant women with COVID-19 who have tested positive in order for spread reduction.
7. Breastfeeding after recovery if tested negative for SIgA and COVID-19 antibody transmission to the growing neonate.

The application and adherence to these recommended and suggested management, preventive and control measures will (a) facilitate epidemic curve flattening and down drifting as well as case fatality mitigation, (b) fetal COVID-19 transmission reduction, and (c) COVID-19 perinatal mortality marginalization.[8] When vaccines become available, adherence to vaccine uptake remains viable and reliable in marginalizing SARS-CoV2 infection among pregnant females who are vaccine eligible.

Maternal Immune System and Fetal Survival

The maternal immune system plays a substantial role in fetal and neonate life, the building block of survival, indicative of the significant role of biological mothers in life course and human existence. While life begins at gametogenesis, the exact moment of conception remains uncertain and not fully understood. This genesis reflects an integration of XX and XY chromosomes for viable oocytes and uterine implantation. However, during gestation, maternal antibodies in the form of immunoglobulin, namely IgM and IgG, are transferred to the fetus via uterine blood perfusion. Maternal transfer of sIgA via breast milk to the neonates, infants and newborns is very substantial and plays a significant role in neurogenesis, gastrointestinal and respiratory tract protection.

With COVID-19 pandemic and subpopulation risk differentials, especially excess case fatality among Blacks/AA and Hispanics, the immunologic response is to acknowledge the contributory role of mothers in antibody transfer, required in marginalized viral replication and compromised virulence and pathogenicity. Today, Mother's Day, we recognize the contribution of all mothers to the survival of the human species. With this contribution, all mothers regardless of social class, race/ethnicity and culture must be equitably valued and recognized in human society.

With the persistent observation of excess mortality of Black/AA infants relative to Whites, this reflection recommends all women of child-bearing age and mothers to be provided with equitable prenatal care, health care access and utilization, social and economic (housing and living conditions) needs in meeting the social determinants of health. This recommendation reflects public health disproportionate universalism in prenatal care and social equity for women of child-bearing age and mothers. With this integrative approach, implying the application of consequentialist public health, minorities who are disproportionately affected by COVID-19 case fatality will benefit, given the life course implication of maternal antibodies' transfer to the fetus during gestation and at breastfeeding.

Questions for Discussion

1. During pregnancy, are oocytes perceived by the maternal immune system as antigen or non-self?

2. Does pregnancy increase viral pathogenic transmission? Explain the immunologic approach in this pathway.
3. Explain how the maternal immune system enhances viral fetal/gestational protection.
4. Describe the subpopulation differentials in fetal interruption during maternal or gestational period SARS-CoV2 infectivity.

Notes

1 Innate and Adaptive Immune Responses in HELLP Syndrome – NCBI". 15 Apr. 2020, https://www.ncbi.nlm.nih.gov/pmc/articles/PMC7174768/. Accessed 12 Nov. 2021.
2 "Relationship between Maternal Immunological Response during …". https://www.ncbi.nlm.nih.gov/pmc/articles/PMC4060291/. Accessed 12 Nov. 2021.
3 "Immunological Tolerance, Pregnancy, and Preeclampsia: The Roles…". 4 Jan. 2018, https://www.ncbi.nlm.nih.gov/pmc/articles/PMC5758600/. Accessed 12 Nov. 2021.
4 "Inflammation and Pregnancy: The Role of the Immune System at the …". https://www.ncbi.nlm.nih.gov/pmc/articles/PMC3078586/. Accessed 12 Nov. 2021.
5 "Why are Pregnant Women Susceptible to COVID-19? An … – NCBI". 19 Mar. 2020, https://www.ncbi.nlm.nih.gov/pmc/articles/PMC7156163/. Accessed 12 Nov. 2021.
6 "Breastfeeding and Caring for Newborns if You Have COVID-19 | CDC". https://www.cdc.gov/coronavirus/2019-ncov/if-you-are-sick/pregnancy-breastfeeding.html. Accessed 12 Nov. 2021.
7 "Pregnant and Recently Pregnant People | CDC". https://www.cdc.gov/coronavirus/2019-ncov/need-extra-precautions/pregnant-people.html. Accessed 12 Nov. 2021.
8 "Effectiveness of the Measures to Flatten the Epidemic Curve of COVID …". 18 Apr. 2020, https://www.ncbi.nlm.nih.gov/pmc/articles/PMC7166106/. Accessed 12 Nov. 2021.

7 SARS-CoV2 (COVID-19) Risk Precipitation and Disproportionate Mortality in African American (AA)/Black Communities

Social Injustice and Gene Expression (Aberrant Epigenomic Modulation)

The unfair and unjust treatment of Blacks/AA especially males by the criminal justice system in the US is clearly indicative of structural and systemic racism, and the dehumanization of life, a primary value.[1,2,3] Historically, and up to the present, communities of color have been treated as inferior to Whites, which is unsupported by any scientific data on cognitive development. Genetically, the variability between Blacks and Whites is <0.1% as observed in DNA sequencing. As one assesses the subpopulation differences in the DNA sequence in the genome, there remains no variances in DNA sequence comparing Blacks/AA and their White counterparts in the US. Such observation is indicative of the shared similarities in DNA sequencing between Black/AA and Whites, and the need for the scientific communities around the world to consider the biological similarities of all persons regardless of sex, race, ethnicity, age or color, rather than to historically (and up to the present) regard one population as inferior to others, namely Blacks/AA.[4] As a world community, slavery remains an inherent ignorance of humanity and with the available data on human values, such a practice has no place in human history and society. However, the observed variance between Blacks and Whites in health outcomes and social adversity is explained by social inequity, such as low education, low income and poverty that interact with the gene, predisposing Blacks to higher morbidity and mortality compared with their White counterparts in the US.[5]

Police Culture: Social Injustice

The recent murder of a 46-year-old George Floyd of Minneapolis, Minnesota, is clearly indicative of the dehumanization of Blacks and the notion of Blacks/AA being inferior to Whites in America. Racial and ethnic minorities are not valued by the criminal justice system, which renders no presumption of innocence upon allegation and arrest. Such a stance violates the fundamental notion of justice in a nation with the rule of law. Any legal system, either criminal or civil, must respect life as a fundamental value and a primary as well as fundamental right. Additionally, all suspects of crime or accused in the violation of public order that prescribes sanction for violators, regardless of race, ethnicity, color and gender, must be presumed innocent until proven guilty by a competent and fair criminal/civil justice system.[6]

Social Adversity and Health Inequities in SARS-CoV2 (COVID-19)

COVID-19 is a clear indication of the unfair and unjust allocation of social, economic and environmental conditions related to health among AA/Blacks. The disproportionate burden of

DOI: 10.4324/9781003424451-7

case morbidity and mortality among Blacks/AA reflects a population deprived of the social determinants for health, and the interaction of these conditions with the gene[7], implying aberrant epigenomic modulation, predisposing this population to impaired wellbeing, increased morbidity and mortality as well as lower life expectancy relative to the White population.

In 2016, *The Nation Health*, a Public Health Newsletter, published a note on police brutality and how such unlawful behaviors by the law enforcement reflects increasing mental illness in the communities of color namely Blacks/AA due to the reckless use of deadly force. This publication made valuable recommendations in police brutality reduction, and the need for public health action, as the vehicle for social injustice. Public health, as a voice of those without voice, has been charged by the World Health Organization to ensure that peace and social justice be sustained in improving human health.[8]

As the public health workforce reflects on the disproportionate burden of deaths in the AA/Black communities in the US, there is a need to reconsider the implication of social inequity in the determinants of health.[9] All scientific communities must respect the value of human life and apply all resources in ensuring that we improve community health through scientific data by encouraging systems of justice all across the world to educate the law enforcement agents on life as a fundamental value regardless of social gradient, race, ethnicity, gender, sexual orientation, income, education, poverty and age.[10] Therefore, failure to do this will render public health and scientific communities incapacitated in addressing human issues for optimal individual and community health actualization.

Unemployment, Social Instability, and SARS-CoV2 Seropositivity and Mortality

While social protest is essential in exercising the second amendment right, such an initiative during the COVID-19 pandemic is scientifically unacceptable as it deviates from social/physical distancing guidelines for viral spread, increasing the transmission of SARS-COV2. The murder of George Floyd, an unarmed Black/AA male by a White police officer in Minneapolis, Minnesota signals a moment of reflection for the nation, requiring a reinvestment in transforming social equity in AA/Black communities in the US.[11]This act of inhumanity should have no place in a nation with the rule of law that is inherent in liberty and justice for all. While we protest this dehumanizing act of the law enforcement officers, we should realize that the unfair treatment of Blacks/AA in this nation is due in part to fear of retaliation from Blacks/AA on dehumanization acts of labor without financial compensation from around 1619, since Blacks during slavery were dehumanized, resulting in post-traumatic enslavement syndrome (PTES) in the White population today. This syndrome generates a phobia among Whites that results in deadly force application by the law enforcement on AA/Blacks. These PTES must be managed with equitable consideration of lives including Black/AA lives as comparable to White lives in the nation. Therefore, as these violent protests continue, we anticipate and model the continued disproportionate impact of COVID-19 on communities of color in the state of Minnesota and other states.

The COVID-19 pandemic should remind us of the disproportionate burden of epidemic and pandemic on populations without health equity, implying the equitable distribution of social, economic and environmental conditions related to health, namely Blacks/AA, American Indians/Alaska Natives and Hispanics. African Americans/Blacks in this pandemic are disproportionately affected by unemployment which translates to social adversity and adverse health outcomes, especially mental illness due to the psychosocial stressors related to unemployability.

The social protest by the Black/AA communities, Hispanics and sensitive Whites in Floyd's murder is necessary as an exercise of the Second Amendment right. However, such protests should be peaceful in line with Rev. Martin Luther King's notion of nonviolent protest, since violence cannot induce peace. With the ongoing protest deviating from the scientific guidelines in COVID-19 transmission, especially social distancing, the scientific community recommends an end to this protest in order to save lives. We as a society, especially scientists, researchers and public health personnel must request justice to be transparent in George Floyd's murder. The third degree murder and manslaughter charges for the police officer in question is unacceptable and, from a procedural criminal justice stance, very unfair and unjust, thus indicative of justice as "unfairness".

The current charge should be changed to first degree murder, and with the inherent "mens rae" and not solely "actus rae" at trial, implying the accused intended to commit the murder, then justice will be served, as there is substantial evidence beyond a reasonable doubt in this case. Additionally, the remaining three police officers involved in this case based on the "actus rea" should be charged in this criminal act. The urgent need to transform these charges will, and should, result in an immediate end to this protest. As a society, if the nation fails to end this protest by ensuring justice through these recommended and appropriate charges, the US will experience increased SARS-CoV2 transmission, not only in the Black/AA communities but other communities taking part in the protest. As a scientific community, we call on the nation, especially the justice department to transform the current violent protest to a peaceful one by objective and criminal law principles/and concept guidelines on charges of this nature, and the subsequent return to social distancing in ending the entire protest. With social distancing implication in SARS-CoV2 transmissibility reduction, if US society fails to address this social instability of persistent protests, SARS-CoV2 exponential transmission will enhance SARS-CoV2 global transmissivity since we all live in a global village.

Questions for Discussion

1. Describe the role of social injustice in SARS-CoV2 transmission differentials by subpopulations.
2. Explain the effect of social instability and lower SES in aberrant epigenomic modulations in excess COVID-19 among racial and ethnic minorities or lower social class.
3. Does police culture in the US and elsewhere result in the exponentiation of viral transmissibility and mortality among racial/ethnic minorities and lower social class?
4. Explain how the disproportionate burden of SARS-CoV2 and COVID mortality impacts health equity.

Notes

1 "Racial and Ethnic Disparities in Years of Potential Life Lost … – MDPI", https://www.mdpi.com/1660–4601/18/6/2921/htm. Accessed 9 Mar. 2022.
2 "Abstracts from the 53rd European Society of Human Genetics …". 1 Dec. 2020, https://www.nature.com/articles/s41431-020-00740-6. Accessed 9 Mar. 2022.
3 "The Sociology of Discrimination – Annual Reviews", https://www.annualreviews.org/doi/10.1146/annurev.soc.33.040406.131740. Accessed 6 Mar. 2022.
4 TESTING AND ASSESSMENT WITH PERSONS & COMMUNITIES …", https://www.apa.org/pi/oema/resources/testing-assessment-monograph.pdf. Accessed 9 Mar. 2022.
5 "Explaining the Black-White Disparity in Preterm Birth – Frontiers". 2 Sep. 2021, https://www.frontiersin.org/articles/10.3389/frph.2021.684207/full. Accessed 9 Mar. 2022.
6 "Waking Up to Whiteness and White Privilege – University of Central …". 7 Oct. 2020, https://www.ucf.edu/news/waking-up-to-whiteness-and-white-privilege/. Accessed 9 Mar. 2022.

7 Racial Disparities in Coronavirus Disease 2019 (COVID-19) …". 1 Mar. 2021, https://pubmed.ncbi. nlm.nih.gov/33221832/. Accessed 9 Mar. 2022.

8 "Why Police Brutality Is a Public Health Issue | SELF". 17 Jun. 2020, https://www.self.com/story/ police-brutality-public-health-issue. Accessed 9 Mar. 2022.

9 "3 The Root Causes of Health Inequity | Communities in Action", https://www.nap.edu/read/24624/ chapter/5. Accessed 9 Mar. 2022.

10 "Understanding Community Policing – Office of Justice Programs", https://www.ojp.gov/pdffiles/ commp.pdf. Accessed 9 Mar. 2022.

11 "Suddenly, Public Health Officials Say Social Justice Matters More …". 4 Jun. 2020, https://www. politico.com/news/magazine/2020/06/04/public-health-protests-301534. Accessed 9 Mar. 2022.

8 Social Injustice and Systemic Racism

Obstacles to COVID-19 Pandemic Global Health Equity Transformation

Social Gradient and Health Outcomes

The World Health Organization (WHO) recommended social justice and peace as necessary conditions for human health, implying social injustice and systemic racism in the perpetually observed racial/ethnic disparities in morbidity and mortality in the US and elsewhere.[1,2,3] While the nation allocates a substantial amount of revenue to the healthcare system, life expectancy and infant mortality do not reflect this investment due, in greater part, to social injustice and systemic racism that perpetuate unequal and inequitable outcomes of care across subpopulations. The US subpopulations that experienced historically and to date systemic and structural racism, namely Blacks/AA and American Indians/Alaska Natives, present with a disproportionate burden of disease including survival disadvantage relative to their White counterparts.[1]

While clinical medicine education and training has traditionally focused on structure (anatomy), function (physiology), alteration of function (pathology) and the restoration of function (pharmacology and surgery), there was no mention of the social determinants of health (SDH) in therapeutics. The current understanding of how psychosocial or social adversity alters human physiology and predisposes to mental and physical illness, signals the social determinants of health as an exposure function of social injustice and systemic racism in morbidity and mortality outcomes.[3,4]

Social Determinants of Health: Structural Racism and Social Injustice Implication

What is SDH, and how does it reflect systemic racism and social injustice? While in medical training, it was stressed that to every physical disease process, there is an emotional reaction. While this observation was and is accurate now, it is quite reliable to claim that, to every emotional disease process or psychosocial adversity, there is a physical illness, which varies depending on adaptation. Social determinants of health simply refers to the opportunity to benefit from the resources necessary for human health including, though not limited to, education, income, occupation, housing, living conditions, food security, peace, safe neighborhood, social justice and racial discrimination.[5] Simply, SDH reflects the social gradient where those with low social hierarchy are more likely to experience low education, unemployment, low median income, unsafe neighborhoods with homicide, decreased access and utilization of the healthcare system and low life expectancy compared to those in the higher social hierarchy. Blacks/AA in the US are socially disadvantaged due to social injustice and systemic racism. There is substantial data that inversely correlates income, education, employment with optimal health outcomes, which provides substantial explanation of the observed health disparities in the US.

DOI: 10.4324/9781003424451-8

Systemic or structural racism reflects the unfair and unjust allocation of economic, social and environment conditions related to human health for Blacks/AA, while the privileged Whites benefit from these resources, and hence higher quality of life, lower morbidity and mortality compared to their Black counterparts.[6] For example, infant mortality is 5.8 per 1,000 among Whites and 13.9 per 1,000 among Blacks, indicative of 139.7% relative difference in infant mortality and 8.1% difference in the absolute measure of IM disparities. Of the industrialized nation in the world, the US ranks the worst in IM, (5.9, 45th). Therefore, addressing systemic racism and social injustice could rank the US 18th globally should the IM in Blacks/AA be comparable to that of the Whites, 5.8 per 1,000.

Health Equity Transformation: COVID-19 Implicit Bias Perspective

Transforming health equity will involve the nation's assessment of the origin of causes and the social gradient pertaining to health, implying the conditions that we live, work and play. The concept of "health-o-graphy" as health and place determines our health which begins from pre-conception, conception, intrapartum event, postpartum, early development, cognitive[7] development, pre-K, high school, college, employment transition, income, and access and utilization of the health care system.

How does systemic racism and social injustice explain racial differences in morbidity and mortality, where Blacks/AA are disproportionately affected compared to their White counterparts? There is no genetic variability between Black/AA and Whites, since the variance in DNA sequence comparing these two racial groups is less than 0.1%. However, what explains the subpopulation variance in disease and mortality outcomes depends on the gene and environment interaction, termed epigenomic modulation. The epigenomic mechanistic process involves the interaction of the gene with the environment that results in DNA methylation at the enhancer region of the gene (C-p-G), influencing gene expression, protein synthesis and cellular functionality. For example, social adversity such as systemic racism provokes social signal transduction of the sympathetic nervous system and the beta-adrenergic receptors involvement in DNA methylation of the glucocorticoid gene receptor (NR3C1), with the hyper DNA methylation of NR3C1 resulting in early life stress and major depressive disorders in adulthood.[8] In effect the aberrant epigenomic modulation associated with systemic racism and social injustice, which could be termed social adversity, has the potential for gene dysregulation, explaining in greater part the Black–White risk differentials in disease outcome, mortality and survival. Therefore, addressing social injustice and systemic racism, reduces social adversity among Blacks/AA, thus enhancing normal epigenomic modulation and decreased morbidity and mortality in this subpopulation of the nation.

The nation requires legislation to end systemic racism and provide equitable opportunity to all Americans regardless of gender, race/ethnicity, sexual orientation, education, income, social class, religion, etc. In addition, the police brutality on AA/Blacks induces mental illness in this population, rendering Blacks/AA with the worst health outcomes in the nation. To address health disparities and transform health equity, we need to address implicit and unconscious bias among law enforcement officers since such dehumanization of Black lives result from systemic racism and post-enslavement traumatic syndrome (PETS),[9] and create a national database for police misconduct as well as train police officers on community policing and life as a primary value.

Since public health is charged with public safety, all public health departments must play a role in ending social injustice and systemic and structural racism in the nation. In addition, since the health of the nation depends on the health status of children, all pediatric healthcare systems must advocate social justice and peace in enhancing the social determinants of health by engaging with policy makers on equitable early pre-K education, and environment that sustains appropriate cognitive development and proficiency in reading skills, high-school graduation, college education and transition to appropriate employment opportunities.[10]

With the significant impact of social injustice and systemic racism on health disparities, transforming health equity requires the provision of equal education, income and healthcare to all Americans. Specifically, we call for public health agencies, institutions and departments, since public health is a collective effort of the society to remain healthy, to end systemic racism and social injustice, because social justice and peace are necessary conditions for human health. As a nation with global leadership initiatives through the CDC, our health ranking in the world depends on how we transform health equity by the narrowing and ultimate elimination of health disparities through clear pathways to ending systemic racism and social injustice.

Questions for Discussion

1. What is the implication of social determinants of health in SARS-CoV2 exponential transmission and infectivity among racial/ethnic minorities and lower social class?
2. Explain how systemic racism adversely impacts epigenomic modulations resulting in excess mortality among some subpopulations in the US and globally.
3. Does implicit bias result in disproportionate burden of SARS-CoV2 infectivity and COVID-19 excess mortality among racial /ethnic minorities and lower social class?

Notes

1 "Structural Racism and Health Inequities – NCBI", https://www.ncbi.nlm.nih.gov/pmc/articles/PMC4306458/. Accessed 9 Mar. 2022.
2 "Promoting Mental Health: Concepts, Emerging Evidence", https://www.who.int/mental_health/evidence/en/promoting_mhh.pdf. Accessed 9 Mar. 2022.
3 "Frontier dialogue consultations on addressing structural racial and …", https://cdn.who.int/media/docs/default-source/documents/gender/frontier-dialogue-unsdg-9-sept.2021.pdf?sfvrsn=bbb8a9e9_5&download=true. Accessed 9 Mar. 2022.
4 "Beyond Health Care: The Role of Social Determinants in Promoting …". 10 May. 2018, https://www.kff.org/racial-equity-and-health-policy/issue-brief/beyond-health-care-the-role-of-social-determinants-in-promoting-health-and-health-equity/. Accessed 9 Mar. 2022.
5 "The Social Determinants of Health: It's Time to Consider the Causes …", https://www.ncbi.nlm.nih.gov/pmc/articles/PMC3863696/. Accessed 9 Mar. 2022.
6 "Structural Racism and Myocardial Infarction in the United States – NCBI", https://www.ncbi.nlm.nih.gov/pmc/articles/PMC4133127/. Accessed 9 Mar. 2022.
7 "The Women's Health Data Book – KFF", https://www.kff.org/wp-content/uploads/2013/01/women-s-health-data-book.pdf. Accessed 9 Mar. 2022
8 "Explaining the Black-White Disparity in Preterm Birth – Frontiers". 2 Sep. 2021, https://www.frontiersin.org/articles/10.3389/frph.2021.684207/full. Accessed 9 Mar. 2022.
9 "Disparities in Health and Health Care: 5 Key Questions and Answers". 11 May. 2021, https://www.kff.org/racial-equity-and-health-policy/issue-brief/disparities-in-health-and-health-care-5-key-question-and-answers/. Accessed 9 Mar. 2022.
10 "The Need to Promote Health Equity - Communities in Action – NCBI", https://www.ncbi.nlm.nih.gov/books/NBK425853/. Accessed 9 Mar. 2022.

9 SARS-CoV2 "Re-emergence" as COVID-19 (2)

Translational Public Health and Immuno-Epidemiologic Response

SARS-CoV2 and Translational Public Health Initiates

While the global pandemic remains the World Health Organization (WHO) initiative in pathogenic microbe mitigation and a return to the pre-pandemic era, this approach requires a translational perspective. With this initiative, national public health systems and the WHO require the collaborative, mutualistic and symbiotic trajectory involving, epidemiologists (population-based data assessment), clinicians/infectious disease experts (diagnosis, treatment, prognosis) and biomedical scientists (immunologic, genetic, epigenetic, genomic, epigenomic, virologic).

SARS-CoV2 Control and Preventive Measures

The current increase in SARS-CoV2 confirmed cases signals national negligence in adherence to control and preventive measures in mitigating this highly contagious viral spread and infectivity.[1,2] These control and preventive measures remain reliable then and currently, namely contact tracing, tracking and testing, physical and social distancing, mask wearing and rigorous hand hygiene. During the month of May 2020, epidemiologic data observed that, unless the nation applies these measures uniformly across all states, there will be a re-emergence of SARS-CoV2, a causative pathogen in COVID-19 disease, severity and mortality. The understanding of viral dynamics is essential in controlling and preventing transmission, however, in the midst of limited transmissibility and infectivity data involving a novel pathogen (disease causing microbe), what is currently known, even though subject to mutation or changes, requires a collective adherence to the infectious disease control protocol. Consequently, this negligence implying US erratic business reopening and the failure of governmental agencies, public and private sector to enforce face mask wearing, appropriate physical and social distancing, rigorous handwashing[3] (disinfectants and soap) as well as the 3Ts – tracing, tracking and testing, results in the observed increase in positive cases, hospitalization overload and increasing morbidity, with anticipated increasing case fatality.

With the clinical manifestation differentials across the COVID-19 patient population, infectious disease, immunologic, epidemiologic and translational public health guidelines require uniform adherence and compliance to control and preventive measures. The SARS-CoV2 mode of transmission clearly illustrates asymptomatic transmission, which implies collective population perception of all persons besides those in the same household as potentially infected individuals, in order to mitigate this spread. Since we, both in the past and currently, perceived all blood samples from HIV-positive individuals to be infective and hence universal precautions were undertaken, we should perceive the current pathogen in the same vein.[4] This perception should result in universal protection where all humans are required by the states, county and

DOI: 10.4324/9781003424451-9

cities to wear face masks. Such a recommendation does not violate our individualism, since collectivism is required in viral spread mitigation and control and not individual rights. The scientific community should acknowledge the implication of collectivism in public health notions, which is what we as a society do to remain healthy.[5] We in the scientific community must mandate mask wearing as a vital public health preventive and control measure for SARS-CoV2.

Besides the public health notion in disease control and prevention as observed in face mask wearing, viral control requires health promotion practices, namely physical and social distancing, as adaptive behavioral modifications.[6] With beaches and businesses reopening (such as gyms, beauty salons, restaurants, etc.), such distancing, even with mask wearing, remains impractical without rigorous hand washing.[7] Therefore, by protecting the health of the nation and ensuring spread mitigation, we can enhance the US economy in the near future. Human health therefore remains a primary value, while the economy is secondary to survival.

SARS-CoV2 Mitigation and Case Reduction Pathways

Translational public health remains a voice for those without a voice, requiring that recommendations be made across all states in the nation on SARS CoV2 control and preventive universalism.[8]

(a) Face mask wearing mandate across all states in the nation and globally.
(b) Reliable and accurate SARS-CoV2 seropositive contact tracing, tracking and testing.
(c) Physical and social distancing within six to nine feet.
(d) Rigorous hand hygiene (disinfecting and washing).

The adherence to these universalisms as observed in some states such as NY, CT, RI, DE, NJ, PA with these control measures, especially face mask wearing, ensures low or no changes in confirmed SARS-CoV2 cases, despite the disproportionate increase in confirmed cases during COVID-19 in these states.[9] Second, since the geographic environment for SARS-CoV2 in the US, un-united transmission control policies remain infeasible in pathogenic microbe prevention and case fatality reduction in the nation.

With public health initiative as a moral responsibility, given human life, the scientific community must engage with the elected officials in ensuring accurate and valid data availability through the CDC for scientific evaluation of these universal recommendations. Therefore, if public health nationally and globally enforce these scientific guidelines across the nation/world regardless of ideology or politics, there remains a feasible opportunity to return the nations to a stable economy, as the world collectively protect lives by enhancing individual productivity across all nations.[10] Further, as the US approaches fall and winter (2020) based on the knowledge of viral dynamics during these seasons, there is an urgent need or emergency response from the scientific community to engage with state, city, county and federal health departments in accessing measures such as universal flu vaccination and chronic disease reliable management in mitigating excess mortalities, which may be synergistic if the nation fails to currently reduce SARS-CoV2 transmission and infectivity.

Questions for Discussion

1. Describe the translational public health pathway in COVID-19 mortality reduction.
2. What are the measures of SARS-CoV2 transmission marginalization?

3. Explain the implication of winter or cold months in viral pandemic upregulation and excess transmission.
4. Does the national application of SARS-CoV2 control and preventive measures result in global mitigation and stabilization?

Notes

1 "Rethinking Herd Immunity and the Covid-19 Response End Game". 13 Sep. 2021, https://publichealth. jhu.edu/2021/what-is-herd-immunity-and-how-can-we-achieve-it-with-covid-19. Accessed 9 Mar. 2022.

2 "Use of Masks to Control the Spread of SARS-CoV-2", https://www.cdc.gov/coronavirus/2019-ncov/ science/science-briefs/masking-science-sars-cov2.html. Accessed 9 Mar. 2022.

3 "Globalization and Infectious Diseases: A Rreview of the Linkages", https://www.who.int/tdr/ publications/documents/seb_topic3.pdf. Accessed 9 Mar. 2022.

4 "Transmission of SARS-CoV-2: Implications for Infection Prevention". 9 Jul. 2020, https://www. who.int/news-room/commentaries/detail/transmission-of-sars-cov-2-implications-for-infection- prevention-precautions. Accessed 9 Mar. 2022.

5 "Strategies for Disease Containment - Ethical and Legal – NCBI", https://www.ncbi.nlm.nih.gov/ books/NBK54163/. Accessed 9 Mar. 2022.

6 "Face Masks During the COVID-19 Pandemic: A Simple Protection …". 13 Jan. 2021, https://www. ncbi.nlm.nih.gov/pmc/articles/PMC7838459/. Accessed 9 Mar. 2022.

7 "Reopening Protocol for Personal Care Establishments: Appendix R". 20 May. 2021, http://publichealth. lacounty.gov/media/Coronavirus/docs/protocols/Reopening_PersonalCare.pdf. Accessed 9 Mar. 2022.

8 "The Find of COVID-19 Vaccine: Challenges and Opportunities", https://www.sciencedirect.com/ science/article/pii/S1876034120307814. Accessed 9 Mar. 2022.

9 "Mask Adherence and Rate of COVID-19 across the United States". 14 Apr. 2021, https://journals. plos.org/plosone/article?id=10.1371/journal.pone.0249891. Accessed 9 Mar. 2022.

10 "Promoting Health Equity – A Resource to Help Communities Address …", https://www.cdc.gov/nccdphp/ dch/programs/healthycommunitiesprogram/tools/pdf/SDOH-workbook.pdf. Accessed 9 Mar. 2022.

10 SARS-CoV2 (COVID-19) Viral Dynamics Control

SARS-CoV2 Mode of Transmission

While viral infectivity, implying transition from the subclinical to clinical phase of infection requires immune responsiveness compromise, case positivity depends on population density, proximity and contact with infected individuals, poor hand hygiene and crowding.[1] SARS-CoV2, the infectious pathogen in COVID-19, had been shown to be transmitted from asymptomatic to uninfected individuals, which renders infectivity control challenging, implying the application of collectivism in mitigating the viral spread. With individualism as relevant as it is to liberty,[2] freedom and autonomy, control of viral spread requires a compromise of such rights in protecting human life through collectivism, implying what we as a society can do collectively to preserve human life – a primary value.[3]

Musculoskeletal function, mainly movement, reflects life. As humans, movement is essential for cardiac conditioning and vitality but such process in an era of pandemic requires individuals to protect the societal interest in preserving life through face mask wearing when in public. With the current approach to school reopening, current data are indicative of increased transmission in college campuses across the nation.[4] Adherence to face mask wearing in such circumstances has a tendency to reduce the viral spread, since asymptomatic individuals could exponentially transmit the virus across diverse populations. Also observed in COVID-19 are clinical manifestations of diversity by age and subpopulations such as race and ethnicity, disability and comorbidities, with less symptom severity and mortality observed among young adults and children.[5] However, the post-diagnostic physiologic consequence of this novel pathogen among children and young adults upon infection is not fully understood.

SARS-CoV2 Control Measures: Physical and Social Distancing, Mask Wearing and Rigorous Hand Hygiene

Physical and social distancing remains a reliable perspective in viral infection control, especially in SARS-CoV2. This distancing reflects low population density with respect to decreased transmission. The nation requires a coordinated effort with six to nine feet distance in school campuses and in every open space including office spacing, schools, places of worship etc.[6] Adherence to these recommendations remains a pathway to case positivity reduction, case fatality mitigation and mortality marginalization in the US. Currently as we observed >1,000 deaths daily in the nation from the mid-August till today, there is a need for all Americans to observe distancing and mask wearing in controlling this viral dynamic.

Relevant to SARS-CoV2 transmission reduction is rigorous hand hygiene. Like most viral pathogens, the pathogenic entry to the portal of transmission such as the nose, eyes or mouth

DOI: 10.4324/9781003424451-10

is significant to transmission.[7] However, hand contact with SARS-CoV2 does not translate to infection unless the hand is applied to the face, compromising the innate immune mechanism – the intact human surface or skin. All Americans must apply disinfectants with Lysol and water upon perceived contact with suspected and non-suspected surfaces for viral survivability prior to face touching.

The increased crowding of beaches, birthday celebrations, garage sales, etc. signals increased spread. Participants in such contacts are required to wear masks, apply six to nine feet distancing, apply an infrared thermometer for individuals prior to participation, and utilize disinfectants before and after contact with other individuals and objects. With the winter season, infectious disease control measures recommend influenza vaccine for all Americans in order to enhance the immune responsiveness and probably the cross-reactive antibodies for SARS-CoV2.[8]

SARS-CoV2 Case Positivity and COVID-19 Mortality Mitigation

The application of these recommendations will facilitate a reduction in case positivity as well as mortality. Therefore, if we fail in applying these recommendations, there is a projected crude and unadjusted model of the total mortality from COVID-19 to be 305,800 lives by the end of the year.[9] Today the total mortality is 191,536 and, by the end of the year, there will be an additional 114,264 lives lost to this pathogenic microbe if the US as a nation does not collectively address these control measures. In addition, the epidemiologic curve has a tendency for mortality reduction which is unlikely, given the size of the nation's population. Therefore, as a notion with public health leadership, we need to collectively address what is scientifically known about SARS-CoV2 transmission and COVID-19 prognosis, case fatality and mortality in returning the society to a SARS-CoV2 transmission mitigated nation by 2021.[10]

While there is some limited knowledge on the measures of SARS-CoV2, as a scientific community and public health officials, there is a moral obligation to protect human life by engaging with communities such as schools, churches, and community centers for adherence to these measures. Specifically, reducing the mortality rate to less than 305,800 lives by the end of the year will require these collective efforts as a nation, namely face mask wearing, physical and social distancing, no crowding and rigorous hand hygiene.[11] Additionally, as a nation with social inequity, populations with the disproportionate burden of COVID-19 should be provided with the disproportionate benefit of contact tracking, tracing, testing and vaccines.[12]

Questions for Discussion

1. Explain the SARS-CoV2 seropositivity tracking and tracing.
2. What are the control and preventive measures in this pathogenic spread?
3. Describe the epidemiologic measures in COVID-19 mortality reduction,
4. Examine physical distancing and SARS-CoV2 spread mitigation.

Notes

1 "Transmissibility and transmission of respiratory viruses – Nature". 22 Mar. 2021, https://www.nature.com/articles/s41579-021-00535-6. Accessed 9 Mar. 2022.
2 "Transition to endemicity: Understanding COVID-19 – NCBI". 24 Sep. 2021, https://www.ncbi.nlm.nih.gov/pmc/articles/PMC8461290/. Accessed 9 Mar. 2022.
3 "What Is a Collectivist Culture? Individualism vs. Collectivism". 23 Feb. 2022, https://www.verywellmind.com/what-are-collectivistic-cultures-2794962. Accessed 9 Mar. 2022.
4 "Wearing Face Masks Strongly Confuses Counterparts in Reading". 25 Sep. 2020, https://www.frontiersin.org/articles/10.3389/fpsyg.2020.566886/full. Accessed 9 Mar. 2022.

5 "To Mask or Not to Mask Children to Overcome COVID-19 – NCBI". 9 May. 2020, https://www.ncbi.
   nlm.nih.gov/pmc/articles/PMC7210459/. Accessed 9 Mar. 2022.
6 "CDC Updates Operational Strategy for K-12 Schools to Reflect New …". 19 Mar. 2021, https://
   www.cdc.gov/media/releases/2021/p0319-new-evidence-classroom-physical-distance.html. Accessed
   9 Mar. 2022.
7 "Community Transmission of SARS-CoV-2 by Surfaces: Risks and …". 6 Jan. 2021, https://pubs.acs.
   org/doi/10.1021/acs.estlett.0c00966. Accessed 9 Mar. 2022.
8 "n for – Rogers-Lowell Chamber of Commerce". https://www.rogerslowell.com/clientuploads/Publi-
   cations/Reopening%20Playbook/RogersLowellOpenforBusiness.pdf. Accessed 9 Mar. 2022.
9 "Estimating Mortality from COVID-19 – WHO | World Health Organization …". 4 Aug. 2020, https://
   www.who.int/news-room/commentaries/detail/estimating-mortality-from-covid-19. Accessed 9 Mar.
   2022.
10 "Understanding Population Health and Its Determinants – NCBI", https://www.ncbi.nlm.nih.gov/
   books/NBK221225/. Accessed 9 Mar. 2022.
11 "Keeping your distance to stay safe – American Psychological Association", https://www.apa.org/
   practice/programs/dmhi/research-information/social-distancing. Accessed 9 Mar. 2022.
12 "Covid-19 Pandemic and the Social Determinants of Health | – The BMJ". 29 Jan. 2021, https://www.
   bmj.com/content/372/bmj.n129. Accessed 9 Mar. 2022.

11 Immune System Senescence in SARS-CoV2 Transmission and COVID-19 Clinical Manifestations, Severity and Complications

SARS-CoV2 Dynamics

COVID-19 remains a viral disease due to SARS-CoV2 infectivity. The entry and replication of viral pathogens in the host requires the compromising of the innate and acquired immune system responsiveness.[1,2,3] Traditionally, as observed with HIV infection, the AIDS causing pathogen, not all exposed to this pathogen presented with the infection – such as married couples and partners during the 1980s and 1990s. This observation validates the role of the immune system response during viral infectivity. Despite this understanding, novel viral pathogens remain challenging in terms of dynamics, implying incubation period/subclinical, clinical manifestation/symptomatic period, asymptomatic manifestations and re-infectivity.[4] Since we are still in search of reliable and accurate data on SARS-CoV2 and COVID-19 transmission, case fatality, and mortality, the nation requires strict adherence to current scientific data in recommending, across all states and US territories, face mask wearing, social and physical distancing regardless of event population density in terms of crowds or clustering (which is not supported by SARS-CoV2 dynamics understanding) and rigorous hand hygiene.[5]

Immunologic Senescence: SARS-CoV2 Risk, Pathogenic Spread and Severity

The notion of immunologic senescence reflects the aging immune system as a biologic decline with advancing age. Biologic and clinico-pathologic data have indicated that, on average, there appears to be a 1% decline in organ-system as a biologic function after age 30, but ophthalmologic changes commence earlier. However, these declines depend on several factors including the immune function as reflected in healthy and balanced nutrients, stress minimization and normal sleep pattern and duration, indicative of a healthy lifestyle.[6]

The biologic decline in aging, manifest as advanced age, signals immune system downregulation that impacts on innate immune system response namely macrophages, neutrophils, monocytes, dendritic cells, interferons as well as the acquired immune response such as T and B lymphocytes as reflected in cytotoxic, helper and suppressor T-cells and the immunoglobulins as antibodies, respectively. As the American population ages, one estimates 20% of the US population will be 65 years or older by 2050.[7] Additionally, as the population ages, with social isolation, rejection, subordination, discrimination and chronic social stress, there is a tendency for the basal transcriptome activities to be influenced via the central nervous system (CNS) control of neural and endocrine process. These CNS changes, as transcriptional dynamics regulation, impact on the immune system response gene such as pro-inflammatory cytokine genes as observed in IL-6, IL-8, TNF, IFN-α and IFN-β, with these interferons as an innate antiviral response in protecting the non-virally infected cells against viral replication.[8]

DOI: 10.4324/9781003424451-11

The aging biologic system with social-environmental adversity as experienced in the aging Black/AA population, predisposed these minorities, especially men, to antiviral response down-regulation by the leucocytes as inferred from the increased elaboration of the conserved transcriptional response to adversity – compromised antiviral immune response gene expression.[9] Specifically, the aging population, with an adverse social environment, is predisposed to transcriptional shift implying decreased activity or the downregulation of the transcriptional factors as observed in interferon response factor, resulting in increased viral replication and symptom amplification, clinical manifestations and organ-system damage and decreased survival. Since the human immune response gene is sensitive to decline in biological functions and social adversity, individuals age 65 and older should apply infectious disease control measures such as face mask wearing, distancing and rigorous hand hygiene in self-protection, thus marginalizing COVD-19 case positivity and fatality.[10]

Geriatrics and Immunologic Senescence

Viral pathogens such as SARS-CoV2 infection among the elderly as a respiratory system manifestation affects multiple organs as it progresses, including the lungs (requiring chest X-ray), clinical evaluation for potential pulmonary thrombosis, renal and cardiovascular function (BP and O_2 blood level concentration). There must be a clear clinical assessment of the elderly in determining if the breathing process improves, as well as lung function, by assessing pneumonia due to viral infiltration and consolidation.[11] Of relevance to organ-system involvement in viral infection, as in COVID-19, are the possibilities for renal, cardiac and cerebrovascular complications, resulting in mortality. Therefore, since being male, overweight, 65 years and older, and comorbidities increase the risk of complication and mortality from COVID-19, clear monitoring of such cases is required for survival advantage.

Individuals with advanced age infected with SARS-CoV2, with moderate to severe symptom manifestations, should be evaluated for elevated temperature, fever as the host response to viral replication, vitals such as O_2 blood level, blood pressure and pulmonary/chest X-ray should be closely monitored. Since the complications of viral COVID-19 involve the renal, cardiac and cerebrovascular systems, these organ-systems must be monitored to ensure survival. Unfortunately, unlike bacterial pathogens that could be addressed by inhibiting bacterial replication and colonization, virus replication requires the host cells for infectivity and must be addressed effectively with vaccines for antibody production and potentiation.[12] Therefore, as the US moves toward vaccine administration, there must be cautious optimism in expecting increased protection prior to community-based administration, after the phase III trial for efficacy and safety. The scientific community and public health officials should collectively advocate no social gathering and crowd restriction in order to stop super spreading of SARS-CoV2 since this pathogen does not discriminate, encourage and stress the importance of face mask wearing as well as rigorous hand hygiene, especially among geriatric patients and the elderly with decreased immune responsiveness – immune senescence.

Questions for Discussion

1. What is immunologic senescence?
2. Explain the implication of aging in increase SARS-CoV2 infectivity.
3. What are the immunologic cells among the elderly that result in increase in SARS-CoV2 infectivity and organ-system complications flowing COVID-19?
4. Discuss the implication of age, obesity, comorbidities and geographic locale in COVID-19 disproportionate burden of mortality.

Notes

1 "Organization and Integration of the Endocrine System – NCBI", https://www.ncbi.nlm.nih.gov/pmc/articles/PMC2128294/. Accessed 9 Mar. 2022.
2 "Aging, Immunity, and COVID-19: How Age Influences the Host …". 12 Jan. 2021, https://www.frontiersin.org/articles/10.3389/fphys.2020.571416/full. Accessed 9 Mar. 2022.
3 "Overview of Immune Response During SARS-CoV-2 Infection". 7 Aug. 2020, https://www.frontiersin.org/articles/10.3389/fimmu.2020.01949/full. Accessed 9 Mar. 2022.
4 Immune Response, Inflammation, and the Clinical Spectrum of …". 16 Jun. 2020, https://www.frontiersin.org/articles/10.3389/fimmu.2020.01441/full. Accessed 9 Mar. 2022.
5 "COVID-19: Epidemiology, Virology, and Prevention – UpToDate". 1 Mar. 2022, https://www.uptodate.com/contents/covid-19-epidemiology-virology-and-prevention. Accessed 9 Mar. 2022.
6 "The Continuum of Aging and Age-Related Diseases: Common – NCBI". 12 Mar. 2018, https://www.ncbi.nlm.nih.gov/pmc/articles/PMC5890129/. Accessed 9 Mar. 2022.
7 "Immunosenescence and Its Hallmarks: How to Oppose Aging …". 25 Sep. 2019, https://www.frontiersin.org/articles/10.3389/fimmu.2019.02247/full. Accessed 9 Mar. 2022.
8 "Social Safety Theory: A Biologically Based Evolutionary Perspective …", https://www.annualreviews.org/doi/10.1146/annurev-clinpsy-032816–045159. Accessed 9 Mar. 2022.
9 "Implication of Spiritual Network Support System in Epigenomic …", https://www.mdpi.com/1660–4601/16/21/4123/htm. Accessed 9 Mar. 2022.
10 "Facing Addiction in America – Surgeon General's Report on Alcohol …". 8 Jul. 2016, https://addiction.surgeongeneral.gov/sites/default/files/surgeon-generals-report.pdf. Accessed 9 Mar. 2022.
11 "Clinical Management of Severe Acute Respiratory Infection (SARI …". 13 Mar. 2020, https://www.who.int/docs/default-source/coronaviruse/clinical-management-of-novel-cov.pdf. Accessed 9 Mar. 2022.
12 "Clinical Characteristics of 5 COVID-19 Cases With Non-respiratory …". 12 May. 2020, https://www.frontiersin.org/articles/10.3389/fped.2020.00258/full. Accessed 9 Mar. 2022.

12 SARS-CoV2 Exponential Spread and COVID-19 Hospitalization, Case Fatality and Mortality

US Pandemic Mitigation and Stabilization Measures Regression

SARS-CoV2 Control and Preventive Measures

The application of accurate, valid and reliable measures in the control and prevention of viral pathogenic spread, infectivity, complications and prognosis is critical in pandemic mitigation and stabilization. With the ongoing case positivity and mortality based on the predictive epidemiologic model, the US had derailed from these control and preventive measures, requiring an immediate response at the national level to control SARS-CoV2 and minimize[1, 2, 3] COVID-19 case fatality and mortality in the US population. With the current surge in more than 50% of states in the nation, this signals an unreliable approach to the collective management of SARS-CoV2 transmission and COVID-19 mortality. Specifically, contact tracing, tracking and testing has not been effectively utilized, in this mitigation, across the nation. Additionally, the "maskless" spread from asymptomatic individuals in large gatherings remains a substantial mechanistic process for the current viral surge, indicative of a national mandate.[4]

Descriptive Epidemiologic Measure: Seasonality and Place (Geographic Locale)

Viral dynamics depend on seasonality, especially the fall and winter months, which enhances sustained replication as well as elevated population density due to proximity and compromised distancing, <6–9 feet. With the enhanced replication of SARS-COV2 in an estimated 50% of the states, namely the Midwestern states, South Dakota, Idaho, Iowa, Wisconsin, seasonality partly explains these waves. Similar observations are expected in the northeast as the cold season evolves. In effect, with increasing viral pathogens during this cold season such as adenovirus, rhinovirus (enterovirus) the most causative pathogen in the common cold, influenza virus, Epstein-Barr virus, etc., SARS-CoV2 has a tendency for enhanced replication.[5]

The simultaneous host colonization by these pathogenic microbes during pandemics has the tendency of lowering immune responsiveness, thus increasing SARS-CoV2 infectivity after exposure. Additionally, the geographic locale, such as counties where rallies were held as well as neighboring counties, indicated increased spread in the nation.[6] Simply, the more cases positivity observed in a population, the more the community spread of the pathogen within such populations. The inability or unwillingness to wear face masks, especially in large crowds, is indicative of exponential spread, since asymptomatic individuals, not tested for case positivity, are SARS-CoV2 super spreaders.

Regardless of a pathogenic microbe, population density with or without rigorous hand hygiene correlates with an increased risk of viral infection. The cold season is indicative of human clustering which explains the increased spread of influenza virus, rhinovirus and adenovirus

DOI: 10.4324/9781003424451-12

Table 12.1 US SARS-CoV2 Seropositivity, COVID-19 Mortality and Case Fatality, October 2020

Period (October)	SARS-CoV2 Seropositivity (n)	COVID-19 Mortality (n)	COVID-19 Case Fatality (per 10,000)
October 15	7,966,634	217,601	273
October 16	8,032,805	218,410	272
October 21	8,275,168	221,083	267
October 22	8,395,100	222,925	266
October 23	8,445,242	223,437	265
October 24	8,697,419	225,067	261
October 25	8,631,158	225,211	261
October 28	8,837,688	227,421	257
October 29	8,927,472	228,439	256
October 30	9,007,298	229,293	255
October 31	9,114,418	230,366	253

Notes and abbreviations: The case fatality proportion was estimated using mortality/case positivity $\times$ 10,000. n = frequency or count.

during the fall and winter months. The states who are characterized by cold winter months and longer duration of the cold season, are more predisposed to increasing community SARS-CoV2 infection due to lower or compromised response to a presenting pathogen or antigen (lowered immunogenicity as pathogenic storm).[7] Despite the observed viral dynamics in SRAS-CoV2 transmissibility, adherence to preventive and control measures remains a reliable and feasible approach to spread reduction and COVID-19 mitigation. With the fall and winter months ahead, SARS-CoV2 community spread reduction will require the nation to mandate face mask wearing while in public and open spaces, six to nine feet physical distance and rigorous hand hygiene. The failure of the nation and the Midwestern as well as Northeastern states to adhere to such mandates may result in excess mortality, greater than the predicted 305,000deaths by December 31, 2020.[8]

Currently, case positivity continues to increase in the nation, implying increased hospitalization, albeit with plateaued mortality (Figure 12.1). While the US constitutes 4.25% of the total global population, the nation represents an estimated 19.9% to 19.3% of the total COVID-19 mortality during October 15 to 30, 2020 (Figure 12.2). In addition, the case fatality rate ranged from 255 to 273 per 10,000 (Figure 12.3). The observed COVID-19 pandemic mitigation strategies have not been achieved in the nation, thus requiring reliable and decisive action in order to protect lives.[9]

Public Health Control and Preventive Measures Reinforcement

Public health remains a collective effort on what we as a society should do to remain healthy. This initiative involves a moral obligation in protecting lives as a primary value. The scientific communities and public health officials, in order to protect lives, enhance the US economy and ensure quality of life – implying aging without disabilities –must remain a voice for those without a voice during this pandemic. With the public health obligation in controlling pandemics, there is a need to consider the following recommendations if we are to lower mortality from COVID-19 by December 2020 and January through March 2021.[10]

Table 12.2 US and Global COVID-19 Case Fatality Rate per 10,000, October 2020

COVID-19 Mortality Period	US Case Fatality Rate	Global Case Fatality Rate
15 October	273	282
16 October	272	288
17 October	270	283
18 October	269	280
19 October	268	279
20 October	268	278
21 October	267	276
22 October	266	273
23 October	265	272
24 October	261	270
25 October	261	269
26 October	259	267
27 October	257	265
28 October	257	264
29 October	256	263
30 October	255	261
31 October	253	260

Notes and abbreviations: The US and global case fatality rate was estimated by number of COVID-19 mortality as well as SARS-CoV2 seropositivity per 10,000. Specifically, mortality rate = number of COVID-19 deaths/SARS-CoV2 cases × 10,000.

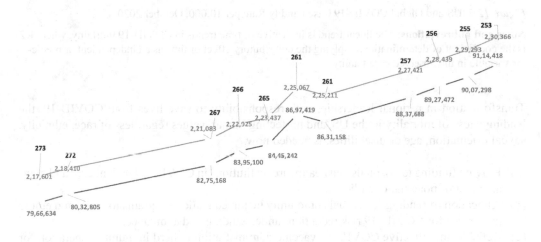

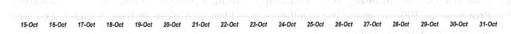

Figure 12.1 US SARS-CoV2 Seropositivity, COVID-19 Mortality and Case Fatality, October 2020

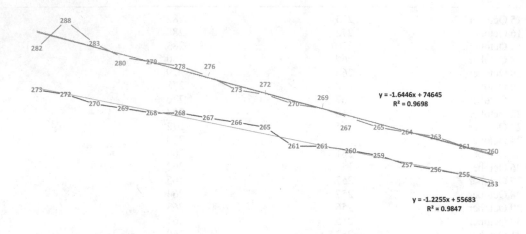

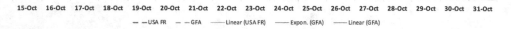

Figure 12.2 US and Global COVID-19 Case Fatality Rate per 10,000, October 2020

Notes and abbreviations: The linear trend is indicative of time trends in COVID-19 mortality, where R2 is the coefficient of determination, implying the contributory effect of time as an independent or predictor variable in the observed case fatality.

Transformation in national leadership, with responsibility to save lives from COVID-19, the leading cause of mortality in the US, and protecting human values regardless of race, ethnicity, sexual orientation, age or disabilities, is needed now.

(a) Provide funding to hospitals and healthcare institutions in COVID-19 patient care and management of potential complications.
(b) Allocation of funding for virtual community health education programs to racial and ethnic minorities for COVID-19 risk reduction, understanding and avoidance.
(c) Reliable and effective COVID-19 vaccine administration in herd immunity generation for community spread reduction and health promotion.
(d) Mandatory use of face masks in public places until SARS-CoV2 spread mitigation and stabilization is achieved.
(e) Establishment of national guidelines and application in contact tracing, tracking and testing.
(f) Provision of PPE in protecting healthcare providers and patients from SARS-CoV2 as a nosocomial viral infection.
(g) Advocating rigorous hand hygiene for all Americans, since viral dynamics implies SARS-CoV2 contact with eyes, mouth and noses, etc. prior to consequential exposure.
(h) Provision of healthy and balanced nutrition to families in need and those with food insecurity for immune system potentiation namely immunoglobulins as glycoproteins.

(i) Advocating remote learning, especially among children and adolescents, for spread reduction.
(j) Ensuring non-evictions for those with economic instability, especially the racial/ethnic minorities and underserved Whites in our nation.
(k) Requiring all Americans, especially the elderly and children with chronic conditions such as diabetes, COPD, asthma or HTN, to be immunized with flu vaccine.
(l) Recommending exercise and a substantial amount of rest via adequate non-REM sleep duration.

Public Health Recommendation: Disease-Specific Leading Cause of Mortality

The COVID-19 pandemic has transformed the US public health experience as the leading cause of mortality in the nation in 2020. Since COVID-19 is an infectious and not a chronic disease but could lead to chronic disease due to organ-system involvement amonge its complications, we as a nation have a moral obligation to act now in saving lives. Therefore, regardless of ideological or political affiliation, we need reliable and responsible leadership in ending this pandemic. As a nation with the rule of law, implying the protection of liberty, freedom and justice, public health, which is a voice for those without a voice, requires a change in national leadership if we are to protect lives and to remain a reliable and accurate machinery for societal and community health improvement. Consequently, public health officials and the scientific community, regardless of political affiliation or ideology, must apply scientific data with effective leadership in addressing and mitigating this COVID-19 pandemic, since the final diagnosis from COVID-19 is mortality, with an estimated lives lost today close to 230,000, which is unacceptable and therefore rejectable, there is an urgent need to transform this pandemic.

Table 12.3 The US Contribution to Global COVID-19 Pandemic Mortality, October 2020

US Mortality Proportion (COVID-19 Global Mortality)	
Period (October, 2020)	*Mortality Proportion (Prevalence/Percentage)*
15 October	19.9
16 October	19.8
17 October	19.8
18 October	19.7
19 October	19.7
20 October	19.6
21 October	19.6
22 October	19.5
23 October	19.5
24 October	19.4
25 October	19.4
26 October	19.3
27 October	19.3
28 October	19.3
29 October	19.2
30 October	19.3
31 October	19.2

Notes and abbreviations: While the US contributes an estimated 4.25% of the global population, the US represents an estimated 19.9% to 19.2% of the total global COVID-19 mortality during October 2020. The mortality proportion or prevalence is estimated by the daily COVID-19 Mortality in the US/Global COVID-19 Mortality x 100.

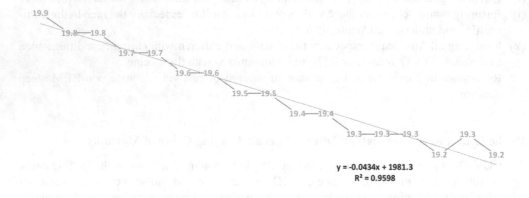

Figure 12.3 The US Contribution to Global COVID-19 Pandemic Mortality, October 2020

Notes and abbreviations: While the US contributes an estimated 4.25% of the global population, the US represents an estimated 19.9% to 19.2% of the total global COVID-19 mortality during October 2020.

Questions for Discussion

1. Explain the non-adherence public health concept in pathogenic microbe, such as SARS-CoV2, control and preventive measures.
2. What are the reliable control and preventive measures in SARS-CoV2 spread?
3. Describe the public health system approach to SARS-CoV2 transmissibility risk reduction nationally and globally by utilizing the WHO requirements.
4. Since the US population represents an estimated 5–6% of the world population, could you explain the predisposing and risk factors to the exponential spread of this viral pathogen in the US?

Notes

1 "Modeling the Effect of Lockdown Timing as a COVID-19 Control …". 8 Feb. 2021, https://www.nature.com/articles/s41598-021-82873-2. Accessed 9 Mar. 2022.
2 "The Territorial Impact of COVID-19: Managing the Crisis Across Levels of Government", https://www.oecd.org/coronavirus/policy-responses/the-territorial-impact-of-covid-19-managing-the-crisis-across-levels-of-government-d3e314e1/. Accessed 9 Mar. 2022.
3 "A Statistical Analysis of the Novel Coronavirus (COVID-19) in Italy and …". 25 Mar. 2021, https://journals.plos.org/plosone/article?id=10.1371/journal.pone.0249037. Accessed 9 Mar. 2022.
4 "The Territorial Impact of COVID-19: Managing the Crisis Across Levels of Government." https://www.oecd.org/coronavirus/policy-responses/the-territorial-impact-of-covid-19-managing-the-crisis-across-levels-of-government-d3e314e1/. Accessed 9 Mar. 2022.
5 "Population Density and Basic Reproductive Number of COVID-19 …". 21 Apr. 2021, https://journals.plos.org/plosone/article?id=10.1371/journal.pone.0249271. Accessed 9 Mar. 2022.

6 "Overview of Immune Response During SARS-CoV-2 Infection". 7 Aug. 2020, https://www. frontiersin.org/articles/10.3389/fimmu.2020.01949/full. Accessed 9 Mar. 2022.

7 "SARS-COV2 Exponential Spread and COVID-19 Hospitalization ...". 31 Oct. 2020, https://www. linkedin.com/pulse/sars-cov2-exponential-spread-covid-19-case-fatality-larry- Accessed 9 Mar. 2022.

8 "'Excess Deaths': How COVID's Broader Toll Highlights Inequity and ...". 4 Jan. 2022, https://www. justhumanproductions.org/articles/excess-deaths-how-covids-broader-toll-highlights-inequity-and-a-need-for-reform/. Accessed 9 Mar. 2022.

9 "COVID Data Tracker Weekly Review | CDC", https://www.cdc.gov/coronavirus/2019-ncov/covid-data/covidview/index.html. Accessed 9 Mar. 2022.

10 "The Future of Public Health Education – NCBI", https://www.ncbi.nlm.nih.gov/books/NBK221190/. Accessed 9 Mar. 2022.

13 SARS-CoV2 (COVID-19) Synergistic Spread

Conjoint Effect of Personal Responsibility, Control/Preventive Measures and Vaccine Effectiveness

SARS-CoV2 Transmission and Global Seasonality

Viral microbe spread and exponential transmission is dependent on temperature in conjunction with population density – as a crowded environment – during winter months. While descriptive epidemiology as an epidemiologic triangle is relevant in viral pathogen control, cold temperature enhances human proximity in a crowded environment, and without face mask wearing and social distancing, pathogenic spread remains exponential.[1] The SARS-CoV2 viral microbe spread reflects increased transmission due to global temperature variance, implying the need for appropriate preventive measures and control.[2]

Environmental Conditions: Climate Changes and Seasonality

The US and global transition into the cold season signals viral spread due to optimum temperature for replication, host population density as well as the US non-adherence to infectious disease control and preventive measures, namely face mask wearing, social and physical distancing, rigorous hand hygiene and feasible lockdown. In the US, the past two weeks is indicative of the deviation from the tenets of viral infection control measures, which resulted in exponential spread of SARS-CoV2, increased hospitalization and excess mortality in some area of the US, namely El Paso, Texas. European nations too have recently experienced increased case positivity but less case fatality and mortality from COVID-19.[3,4] While recovery from COVID-19 had been enhanced thanks to a unified and collective effort at both the treatment and management level to apply the data from the onset of pathogenic clinical features and manifestations for symptom management, the outcome in terms of comorbidities and complications thereafter is not fully understood, requiring cautious optimism in the approach towards COVID-19 therapeutics.

SARS-CoV2 Transmissibility and Host Factor

Viral dynamics, such as in SARS-CoV2, requires the host cell for replication and infection, which is contingent on immune responsiveness in allowing access to the host system and subsequent disease manifestation from asymptomatic, termed subclinical, to symptomatic, implying clinical manifestations.[5] The immunologic dogma is indicative of innate and/or adaptive immune system compromise prior to symptom manifestation or infection, reflecting progression from subclinical to clinical stage of a disease.[6] Specifically, not all exposed to SARS-CoV2 will be infected or develop COVID-19, however, the more contagious a pathogenic microbe is, the higher the risk of infection – as in SARS-CoV2. With this pathogen, there is a need for personal responsibility in reducing the spread or transmission, given the limited knowledge of

DOI: 10.4324/9781003424451-13

this pathogenic pathophysiology and potential organ-system involvement following recovery.[7] As individuals, we must protect ourselves from the transmission, implying "herd protection", where community spread decreases if we assume this as a moral responsibility.

SARS-CoV2 Dynamics, Control and Preventive Measures

There are substantial data on mask wearing and SARS-Cov2 transmission reduction. Specifically, viral pathogenic spread identified through aerosol as well as airborne requires spread mitigation via nose and mouth covering, and hand or body surface contact restriction with the viral pathogen.[8] With the current exponential spared of this pathogen and the anticipated case fatality, given the increase in hospitalization across all epicenters today, face mask wearing remains a national and global mandate.[9] This initiative will mitigate this pandemic both nationally and globally. With the mortality rate today (November 15, 2020) in the US being 2,252 per 100,000, and the US contributing to 21% of the global COVID-19 mortality, we need to have a notional leadership in addressing this pandemic. As a civilized society, there must be an acknowledgment of collectivism over individualism when it comes to pandemics.[10] Therefore, mandatory face mask wearing during the spread of a contagious pathogen that impacts on human life as a primary value, does not infringe on our constitutional right of individual autonomy, liberty and freedom.

Physical and social distancing had been shown to reduce the spread of viral pathogens such as SARS-Cov2.[11] The modification of such behaviors during a pandemic has a potential benefit in protecting lives and ensuring optimal health of the community. Social distancing even with mask wearing is a recommended approach to viral transmission mitigation. While average data in terms of distancing claims 6 feet apart, there is bio-engineering data that recommend 9–12 feet apart in transmission reduction and spread mitigation. The application of these distancing measures, especially in the context of non-mandatory mask wearing, has a substantial impact on viral spread reduction.[12] However, given space restrictions in terms of office space, grocery stores space, etc., there is a need to nationally and globally mandate face mask wearing in SARS-Cov2 spread reduction during this cold and flu season. Therefore, the nation's non-adherence to such measures will result in a predictive model with 312,238 deaths by December 31, 2020, which is indicative of an increasing positive trend based on the October 2020 predictive model with an estimated 305,000 deaths by the end of the year.

Upon the mRNA vaccine uptake, the Pfizer/Modena vaccine as mRNA penetrates the human cells, resulting in spike protein elaboration that recognizes the immune system, resulting in lymphocyte activation and IL-4 enhancement of specific antibody elaboration for SARS-CoV2. With exposure to SARS-CoV2, the specific antibody binds to this viral pathogen inhibiting its replication, implying no infectivity or clinical manifestations.

SARS-Cov2 mRNA versus traditional vaccine reflects a novel vaccine technology that utilizes the genetic sequence of SARS-CoV2 in subsequent antibody production.[13] Unlike traditional vaccines which utilize toxoids, implying the inactivated dose of a pathogenic microbe in disease causation, this novel mRNA vaccine generates a "spike" protein by the host in vaccinated individuals. The viral mRNA which carries the instruction for the cells to generate this "spike" protein as a new coronavirus, that triggers the host to initiate immunologic defense, namely specific antibody production has been shown in several settings to be efficacious and safe.[14] With the 90% efficacy of this vaccine, it is highly likely that herd immunity will be achieved, which raises the issue on the feasibility of vaccination. The questions remain: will the vaccine be effective for racial/ethnic minorities namely Blacks/AA, American Indians/Alaska Natives and Hispanics if these subpopulations were not part of the phase III clinical trial? Were children and the elderly, including those with comorbidities, namely HTN, CVDs, etc. as well as pregnant women, part of this phase III trial? If the trial involved these subpopulations, especially racial/ethnic minorities, we need to apply disproportionate benefit in rendering immediate access to subpopulations, given the disproportionate burden of case fatality and mortality among those populations in the US.

Epidemiologic and Public Health Response and Recommendation

With thanksgiving approaching, and the lack of national leadership in applying reliable and accurate scientific data in these viral control and preventive measures, we in the scientific community and public/societal health officials/researchers would like to recommend these guidelines if we are to experience reduction in daily COVID-19 mortality, implying <312,328 deaths by December 2020:

- Application of personal responsibility in adhering to all the recommended public health measures in SARS-Cov2 spread reduction and mitigation.
  - These measures ensure individuals, families and communities protection, resulting in "herd immunity".
- Utilization of face masks outdoors and indoors, especially during thanksgiving with families and friends/colleagues.
- Application of –six to nine feet social and physical distancing indoors and outdoors, implying large crowd avoidance and human clustering at bars, pools, beaches, etc.
- Rigorous hand hygiene that involves hand disinfectant application and, immediately thereafter, hand washing with soap and water.
- Contact tracking, tracing and testing, which enhances control of SARS-Cov2 spread by asymptomatic individuals.
- Rational, reliable and realistic states, counties and cities lockdown during these winter months as applicable, which had been shown to be effective in transmission reduction in Belgium, Western Europe.
- Immediate vaccination of the communities at increased risk of SARS-Cov2 transmission and those that are currently disproportionately affected by COVID-19 mortality, namely Blacks/AA and Hispanics. This will ensure a disproportionate benefit of this vaccine for these communities, hence herd immunity.

In summary, adherence to these recommendations, especially in the midst of marginalized public health leadership during the COVID-19 pandemic, and the local, county and state public health departments' surveillance and monitoring of this pathogenic spread, will assist substantially in mortality reduction across all subpopulations, thus rendering health equity during the COVID-19 pandemic both in the nation and globally.

Questions for Discussion

1. Differentiate between mRNA and toxoid vaccine. Explain the advantage and disadvantage of mRNA vaccine.
2. Does community adherence to vaccine uptake enhance community herd immunity?
3. Does human gathering (crowd) during events, such as thanksgiving in the US, increase the SARS-CoV2 transmission, resulting in novel variants or strains as anti-genic subtype elaboration for continuous viral survivability?
4. Explain how environmental temperature, as well as human population density, enhances viral spread.

Notes

1 "Environmental Factors Affecting the Transmission of Respiratory Viruses", https://www.ncbi.nlm.nih.gov/pmc/articles/PMC3311988/. Accessed 9 Mar. 2022.

2 "The Potential Future of the COVID-19 Pandemic: Will SARS-CoV-2 …". 3 Mar. 2021, https://jamanetwork.com/journals/jama/fullarticle/2777343. Accessed 9 Mar. 2022.

3 "Use of Artificial Intelligence in Infectious Diseases – NCBI". 13 Mar. 2020, https://www.ncbi.nlm.nih.gov/pmc/articles/PMC7153335/. Accessed 9 Mar. 2022.

4 "Coronavirus Disease (COVID-19) Weekly Report – WHO | World …". 12 Oct. 2020, https://www.who.int/docs/default-source/coronaviruse/situation-reports/20201012-weekly-epi-update-9.pdf. Accessed 9 Mar. 2022.

5 "Severe Acute Respiratory Syndrome Coronavirus 2 (SARS-CoV-2)". 18 Apr. 2020, https://www.ncbi.nlm.nih.gov/pmc/articles/PMC7165108/. Accessed 9 Mar. 2022.

6 "Adaptive Immunity to SARS-CoV-2 and COVID-19 – NCBI". 12 Jan. 2021, https://www.ncbi.nlm.nih.gov/pmc/articles/PMC7803150/. Accessed 9 Mar. 2022.

7 "COVID-19: Current Understanding of its Pathophysiology, Clinical …", https://pmj.bmj.com/content/97/1147/312. Accessed 9 Mar. 2022.

8 "Updated – CDC has Updated Guidance". https://www.cdc.gov/coronavirus/2019-ncov/hcp/infection-control-recommendations.html. Accessed 9 Mar. 2022.

9 "COVID-19 Vaccination and Testing; Emergency Temporary Standard". 5 Nov. 2021, https://www.federalregister.gov/documents/2021/11/05/2021–23643/covid-19-vaccination-and-testing-emergency-temporary-standard. Accessed 9 Mar. 2022.

10 "The Role of Collectivism–Individualism in Attitudes Toward – Frontiers". 28 Oct. 2021, https://www.frontiersin.org/articles/10.3389/fpsyg.2021.600826/full. Accessed 9 Mar. 2022.

11 "Coronavirus, Social and Physical Distancing and Self-Quarantine". 15 Jul. 2020, https://www.hopkinsmedicine.org/health/conditions-and-diseases/coronavirus/coronavirus-social-distancing-and-self-quarantine. Accessed 9 Mar. 2022.

12 "Identifying Airborne Transmission as the Dominant Route – PNAS", https://www.pnas.org/content/117/26/14857. Accessed 9 Mar. 2022.

13 "SARS-CoV-2 Vaccines in Development | Nature". 23 Sep. 2020, https://www.nature.com/articles/s41586-020-2798-3. Accessed 9 Mar. 2022

14 "Immune-mediated Approaches Against COVID-19 – Nature". 13 Jul. 2020, https://www.nature.com/articles/s41565-020-0732-3. Accessed 9 Mar. 2022.

14 SARS-CoV2 Vaccine versus Vaccination

Immunologic Durability and Community Disproportionate Benefit in the United States and Globally

Vaccines or Vaccination?

While vaccines require the scientific community application of data on the mechanism of action, pharmacokinetics and dynamics, safety, efficacy, effectiveness and durability,[1,2,3] vaccination implies community desirability in its administration[4] and the available resources such as dosage and healthcare providers' administration of the US Federal Drug and Administration (FDA) approved vaccines. As the current mortality rate from COVID-19 is increasing daily with positive exponential trends, vaccine effectiveness in preventing COVID-19 development after exposure to SARS-CoV2 is necessary in reversing COVID-19 as the leading cause of death both in the US today and globally.

SARS-CoV2 Vaccine: Mechanism of Action

The current data on the application of novel technology in SARS-CoV2 vaccine development, implying the utilization of SARS-CoV2 genetic material, namely SARS-CoV2 mRNA for subsequent SARS-CoV2 antibody production, reflects efficacy and safety.[5] The observed safety of mRNA vaccine is due to the transition from traditional vaccine development with toxoids, as an altered pathogenic microbe, and its subsequent administration for antibody generation in neutralizing an invading specific pathogen such as SARS-CoV2.[6] However, the durability of this novel mRNA vaccine in terms of antibody sustainability remains to be achieved, and if not, vaccination will be seasonal in protecting individuals and communities from future SARS-CoV2 pathogenic microbes.

SARS-CoV2 Vaccine Uptake, Hesitancy and Benefits

Vaccination requires the administration of vaccines considered by the scientific community in the phases of the trial to be safe and efficacious.[7] The current data based on the phase III trial, reflect safety and efficacy but data remain to be shared on subpopulation responses such as racial/ethnic, age, sex, comorbidity, sample size, response percentage and adverse effects. In effect, given the homogeneity of response in terms of the overall population efficacy of >90%, there is a scientific concordance in its recommendation for all communities in the US, including Blacks/AA, Hispanics and American Indians (AI)/Alaska Natives (AN) to be vaccinated. Also, the elderly, given immunologic senescence or declined immune responsiveness, children with chronic conditions and individuals with comorbidities should be prioritized in this vaccine administration.[8]

DOI: 10.4324/9781003424451-14

As humanity is required to maintain an appointment with history, the Black community has remained skeptical, and continues to do so with vaccines because of the *treponema pallidum* (syphilis) experiment.[9] The US ublic health service initiated an experiment in a southern state (Macon County, Alabama) to observe untreated syphilis. This study involved 600 Black men as subjects with 399 as cases with untreated conditions. Such a practice was, and remains, unethical since ethical studies cannot, and should not, enroll individuals with clinically diagnosed conditions in a study without treatment. Allowing such practices to continue is to render public health, medicine and societal efforts for health and well-being unattainable, since public health is what we all do as a society to remain healthy. We in the scientific community must establish the trust and confidence of the Black community in ensuring that they remain a part of the US community for herd immunity attainment in COVID-19 by commitment to receiving this safe and efficacious mRNA SARS-Cov2 vaccine.[10] The healthcare providers in this vaccine administration must mirror the recipients, requiring the prioritization of this vaccine among Blacks/AA, Hispanics and AI/AN healthcare providers in enhancing trust and confidence. Therefore, given the current mandatory ethical practice in public health and medicine, Blacks/AA must have confidence in the system in terms of vaccine administration and receive the current mRNA vaccine for herd immunity.[11]

With the exponential increase in SARS-Cov2 transmission, there is a need for a collective responsibility in enhancing herd immunity in the US population, especially, the subpopulations disproportionately affected by this pandemic, namely Blacks/AA, American Indians and Hispanics. Additionally, the current new strain of SARS-Cov2 pathogen, although not more virulent relative to the initial strain in terms of antigenicity, is highly transmissible, requiring an urgent mitigation of its spread.[12] Therefore, despite this epitope and antigenic variance, the current mRNA vaccine is uni-vocally and collectively recommended, which might protect against the current strain, given antigenic cross-reactivity. With the overall benefits relative to risk of this novel vaccine, we must ensure that "risk culture" and "healthism" that reflect individual autonomic and health perception, respectively, should not be the building block for vaccine hesitancy (VH).

With mRNA vaccine for SARS-Cov2 immunity, in terms of antibody production to prevent infectivity and symptom manifestation following exposure to this pathogenic microbe, we must weigh between the risk and benefits.[13] While vaccine resistance and vaccine opposition had been used to describe vaccine reluctance and refusal, VH reflects the World Health Organization's characterization as the delay in acceptance or refusal of vaccines despite availability of vaccination services. With medicine and public health not conceived as an exact science, the available data on mRNA vaccine is indicative of its safety and efficacy. However, like the flu vaccine, the public requires applied scientific data on the expectation of this mRNA in terms of COVID-19 manifestations.[14] Specifically, the flu vaccine prevents infectivity, symptom manifestations and severity, which is anticipated from this SARS-Cov2 vaccine.[15] Consequently, it is highly unlikely and scientifically misleading to the public to embrace the notion of "absolute immunity" following vaccine acceptance. With the benefits in this context outweighing the risk, vaccine hesitancy must be completely discouraged through education of the population with a risk culture and Blacks/AA to receive this vaccine for individual, community health and survival benefits.[16]

Currently, the populations most disproportionately affected by COVID-19 are Blacks/AA and Hispanics. Blacks/AA with essential or primary hypertension (HTN) and other comorbidities are disproportionately burdened both nationally and within the communities of color, in terms of SARS-Cov2 case positivity, case fatality and mortality risk.[17] Unlike the White population where HTN is driven less by volume loading and depletion, Blacks are more hypertensive due to excess volume loading and minimal volume depletion, requiring the use of Fosinopril/ HCT, an angiotensin converting enzyme (ACE) inhibitor and angiotensin receptor blocker (ARB) drugs in HTN treatment and management.[18] Specifically, SARS-CoV-2 interfaces with the renin-angiotensin-aldosterone system (RAAS) through ACE2, which modulates RAAS effects as well as serves as a primary receptor for SARS-Cov2.[19] The interaction between this pathogenic microbe and ACE2 is explained in part by RAAS inhibition, transforming ACE2 expression, and therefore rendering SARS-Cov2 virulent among Blacks/AA in the US. Since essential or primary hypertension as a chronic disease is not curable but is treatable, and Blacks/ AA are more predisposed to this condition due to aberrant epigenomic modulation as a result of stressful environment, structural racism, subordination, low SES, marginalized social hierarchy and disadvantaged neighborhood environment, and not genomic variance, we in the scientific community and public health should encourage Blacks/AA to receive this vaccine for herd immunity and mortality reduction.[20] For example a recent study by Holmes L Jr *et al.* observed 74% case positivity among Blacks/AA in Washington DC during the last week in November and the first week in December 2020, implying the disproportionate burden of SARS-Cov2 transmission, given the 49% population size of this subpopulation (Blacks/AA). Additionally, relative to Whites, Blacks/AA were four times as likely to die from COVID-19 during this period. Further, relative to Whites, Hispanics were 25% more likely to die.[21] These findings remain to encourage the communities of color, namely Blacks/AA, to be less reluctant to receive this vaccine, which is a collective decision that transcends individualism and individual autonomy during pandemics.

While an appointment must be kept with history with respect to the nation's public health *treponema pallidum* Tuskegee experimental study of the 1930s, there had been significant changes in the application of such unethical research to observe the natural history or course of a disease. The WHO, CDC and other government health organizations cannot, and should not, be involved in such unethical studies, which is not only immoral but scientifically degrading, since reliable and accurate data are required in human society transformation. We in the Black communities must develop confidence in this mRNA vaccine, which is based on our limited immunologic knowledge of its durability and SARS-Cov2 neutralization for enhanced immune complex development.[22]

Since Blacks/AA are disproportionately burdened by SARS-Cov2 transmission and COVID-19 mortality, the states, counties and cities in a nation with the rule of law must provide this population with a disproportionate benefit of this vaccine including the timely administration of the second dosage for enhanced immunogenicity. Therefore, to increase confidence and trust for this vaccine acceptance among Blacks/AA, this review, as a descriptive epidemiologic initiative, recommends the following:

1. Education of the communities of color on data that reflect the disproportionate burden of SARS-Cov2 transmission and COVID-19 mortality among Blacks/AA, AI/AN as well as Hispanics.
2. Education on the safety and effectiveness (phase IV) of this vaccine in the Black/AA, AI/AN and Hispanic communities, healthcare providers of color, as well as Blacks/AA ministers in faith-based communities.
3. Prioritization of vaccine administration among Black/AA healthcare providers and the publicity in such receipt.
4. Involvement of blacks/AA in vaccine administration to Blacks/AAs in hospitals and community health settings for trust and confidence.

Epidemiologic and Public Health Recommendation

With the current disproportionate burden of COVID-19 mortality, case fatality, complications and comorbidity from SARS-CoV2 (COVID-19) among Blacks/AA, Hispanics and AI/AN, there is a need for the disproportionate adminstration of this vaccine in these subpopulations.[23] The scientific community and public health agencies must request the nation to prioritize this vaccine in populations with the disproportionate burden of this pandemic. Applying this recommendation has two fundamental values, namely herd immunity in these communities of color and marginalized SARS-Cov2 in all communities across the nation and globally.[24] Therefore, failure to advocate, stress and emphasize this recommendation will render the initiative in mitigating this pandemic unachievable.

Questions for Discussion

1. Describe the concepts "vaccine" and "vaccination" and their implications in SARS-CoV2 transmission reduction and COVID-19 mortality marginalization.
2. Examine the Black/AA experience with *treponema pallidum* (syphilis) and the implication in vaccine uptake in the US. What will you consider as public health recommendations in SARS-CoV2 vaccine uptake among this population in the US?
3. Explain why the Black populations in the US are more predisposed to essential or primary hypertension compared to their White counterparts and the implication of this as a comorbidity in the disproportionate burden of COVID-19 mortality in this population.
4. Examine the public health initiative in the disproportionate burden of COVID-19 among Blacks/AA and the guidelines in addressing this burden in future pandemic.
5. Explain the disproportionate universalism in COVID-19 mortality marginalization in the racial/ethnic communities.

Notes

1 "Vaccines Need Not Completely Stop COVID Transmission to Curb …". 18 Jan. 2021, https://www.scientificamerican.com/article/vaccines-need-not-completely-stop-covid-transmission-to-curb-the-pandemic1/. Accessed 9 Mar. 2022.
2 "How to Protect Yourself & Others | CDC", https://www.cdc.gov/coronavirus/2019-ncov/prevent-getting-sick/prevention.html. Accessed 9 Mar. 2022.
3 "Impact of Vaccines; Health, Economic and Social Perspectives". 14 Jul. 2020, https://www.frontiersin.org/articles/10.3389/fmicb.2020.01526/full. Accessed 9 Mar. 2022.
4 "WHO Preferred Product Charactcristics and Clinical Development …", https://cdn.who.int/media/docs/default-source/malaria/ppcs-etc/who-ucn-gmp-2021.03-eng.pdf?sfvrsn=b07d12ef_10. Accessed 9 Mar. 2022.
5 "SARS-CoV-2: Structure, Biology, and Structure-Based Therapeutics …". 25 Nov. 2020, https://www.frontiersin.org/articles/10.3389/fcimb.2020.587269/full. Accessed 9 Mar. 2022.
6 "What are mRNA Vaccines and How do they Work? – MedlinePlus", https://medlineplus.gov/genetics/understanding/therapy/mrnavaccines/. Accessed 9 Mar. 2022.
7 "Ensuring the Safety of Vaccines in the United States | CDC", https://www.cdc.gov/vaccines/hcp/conversations/ensuring-safe-vaccines.html. Accessed 9 Mar. 2022.
8 "Tackling Immunosenescence to Improve COVID-19 Outcomes and …". 1 Nov. 2020, https://www.thelancet.com/journals/lanhl/article/PIIS2666–7568(20)30011-8/fulltext. Accessed 9 Mar. 2022.
9 "Vaccine Development for Syphilis – NCBI". 18 Jul. 2016, https://www.ncbi.nlm.nih.gov/pmc/articles/PMC5513191/. Accessed 9 Mar. 2022.
10 "Tuskegee Syphilis Experiment – An Overview | ScienceDirect Topics", https://www.sciencedirect.com/topics/medicine-and-dentistry/tuskegee-syphilis-experiment. Accessed 9 Mar. 2022.
11 "Medicare and Medicaid Programs; Omnibus COVID-19 Health Care …". 5 Nov. 2021, https://www.federalregister.gov/documents/2021/11/05/2021–23831/medicare-and-medicaid-programs-omnibus-covid-19-health-care-staff-vaccination. Accessed 9 Mar. 2022.

12 "The Origins and Potential Future of SARS-CoV-2 Variants of Concern …". 23 Jun. 2021, https://www.ncbi.nlm.nih.gov/pmc/articles/PMC8220957/. Accessed 9 Mar. 2022.

13 "COVID-19: Epidemiology, Virology, and Prevention – UpToDate". 1 Mar. 2022, https://www.uptodate.com/contents/covid-19-epidemiology-virology-and-prevention. Accessed 9 Mar. 2022.

14 "A Study to Evaluate Efficacy, Safety, and Immunogenicity of mRNA …", https://clinicaltrials.gov/ct2/show/NCT04470427. Accessed 9 Mar. 2022.

15 "Interim Clinical Considerations for Use of COVID-19 Vaccines | CDC", https://www.cdc.gov/vaccines/covid-19/clinical-considerations/covid-19-vaccines-us.html. Accessed 9 Mar. 2022.

16 "Exploring the Continuum of Vaccine Hesitancy Between African …". 29 Dec. 2016, https://www.ncbi.nlm.nih.gov/pmc/articles/PMC5309123/. Accessed 9 Mar. 2022.

17 "The Impact of COVID-19 on African American Communities in the …", https://www.ncbi.nlm.nih.gov/pmc/articles/PMC7702977/ . Accessed 9 Mar. 2022.

18 "First-line Drugs for Hypertension – NCBI", https://www.ncbi.nlm.nih.gov/pmc/articles/PMC6513559/. Accessed 9 Mar. 2022.

19 "Renin–Angiotensin–Aldosterone System Inhibitors in Patients with …". 30 Mar. 2020, https://www.ncbi.nlm.nih.gov/pmc/articles/PMC7121452/. Accessed 9 Mar. 2022.

20 "The Link Between Structural Racism, High Blood Pressure and Black …". 15 Apr. 2021, https://www.heart.org/en/news/2021/04/15/the-link-between-structural-racism-high-blood-pressure-and-black-peoples-health. Accessed 9 Mar. 2022.

21 "SARS-Cov2 Vaccine Hesitancy among Blacks/AAs – LinkedIn". 20 Dec. 2020, https://www.linkedin.com/pulse/sars-cov2-vaccine-hesitancy-among-blacksaas-novel-larry-. Accessed 9 Mar. 2022.

22 "Frontiers | SARS-CoV-2 mRNA Vaccines Elicit Different Responses …". 27 Sep. 2021, https://www.frontiersin.org/articles/10.3389/fimmu.2021.728021/full. Accessed 9 Mar. 2022.

23 "Why are Blacks Dying at Higher Rates from COVID-19? – Brookings". 9 Apr. 2020, https://www.brookings.edu/blog/fixgov/2020/04/09/why-are-blacks-dying-at-higher-rates-from-covid-19/. Accessed 9 Mar. 2022.

24 "A Plan to Work with Communities of Color Toward COVID-19 …". 6 Feb. 2021, https://www.centerforhealthsecurity.org/our-work/pubs_archive/pubs-pdfs/2021/20210209-CommuniVax-national-report.pdf. Accessed 9 Mar. 2022.

15 "COVIDMAS" and SARS-CoV2 (COVID-19) Pandemic Attenuation

Emerging New Strain (Antigenic Subtypes) and Subpopulations Obstacles to Vaccination

SARS-CoV2 Exponential Transmission: Christmas Risk and Epigenomic Modulations

The increase in crowd or family gathering, especially given the new SARS-CoV2 variant, is indicative of the observed SARS-CoV2 case positivity in the US and other nations.[1,2,3] Viral dynamics, as observed earlier, involve population density, implying the closer we are, with limited space and distancing, the higher the likelihood and probability of exponential spread of this viral pathogen.[4] A virus, such as SARS-CoV2, is a coat of protein wrapped around genetic code such as DNA or RNA, and in the case of SARS-CoV2, an RNA, implying that viral microbes are not cells or living cellular organisms, thus requiring host cells for replication and survival.[5] With this new variant, which is a normal process of viral replication and survivability within the host cell, there is no data to support its extreme virulence relative to the initial SARS-CoV2, despite its highly contagious and transmission dynamics compared to the initial strain or variant.[6] Subsequently, viral mutation occurs as the virus is replicating, implying viral survival through mutation, which is a random act, rather than a deliberate act by the virus to enhance survivability.[7]

Novel Variant and Population Density

The observed nature of the highly transmissible pattern of this new variant signals the public health agencies and individual's application of extreme and aggressive preventive and control modalities in SARS-CoV2 spread reduction, relative to the initial strain.[8] The US, as a nation, must apply these current data on this new variant, and mandate mask utilization in family gathering, outside small crowds, outside environment or public and in places of worship as COVIDMAS, rather than Christmas this week. Very significant today is face mask wearing given the mode of transmission of SARS-CoV2 and the new variant or strain as well as rigorous hand hygiene. With a collective and rational approach to mitigating this spread, we can turn the clock around on SARS-Cov2 case positivity and COVID-19 mortality.[9]

Epidemiologic Predictive Modeling: Deaths and Case Fatality

Epidemiologic models for mortality prediction depend on the assumptions in model specification and modeling. Epidemiologists did predict more than 300,000,00 deaths by December 31, 2020. One's model of October 2020 predicted 312,283 deaths by the last day of December 2020, however, since this model did not incorporate the Christmas celebration in its assumption, the current COVID-19 mortality (330,279 deaths) exceeds our predictive model. The currently observed COVID-19 mortality in LA, with an estimated six deaths every hour, implying 44 deaths

DOI: 10.4324/9781003424451-15

every 24 hours is indicative of the need to apply the "limited scientific" data in such a setting to reduce SARS-Cov2 infectivity and COVID-19 mortality.[10] The ability to consider and address crowd gathering and face mask application or use during family gathering, especially in this upcoming New Year celebration, as a healthful new year is relevant in rounding the clock or mitigating global pandemics.[11]

With the efficacy, effectiveness and safety of this current SARS-Cov2 mRNA vaccine, and the acceptance of the population being disproportionately burdened by COVID-19 mortality, such as Blacks/AA, Hispanics and American Indians, we in the scientific community must ensure that access translates to utilization of the vaccine.[12] Communities of color, despite access to care in general, are unable to utilize optimal care and preventive health services due to language translation obstacles for Hispanics and transportation access to Blacks/AA, Hispanics and American Indians in care utilization.[13] The locations or geographic sites for SARS-CoV2 mRNA vaccination in communities of color, mainly Blacks/AA and American Indians, hinder the vaccination administration and acceptance process, implying an urgent need for vaccination access and utilization.[14] We must provide transportation for those without these means to receive this safe and effective vaccine.

Spread Marginalization and Public Health Recommendations

As human society experiences this exponential spread, the public health and scientific communities must recommend to all Americans, and the global village, regardless of constitutional rights and individual autonomy, the following measures of control and prevention:

- Consistent face mask wearing in protecting ourselves and others from infection.
- Social and physical distancing, six to nine feet.
- Rigorous hand hygiene.
- Healthy lifestyle for immune system potentiation (adequate rest, non-REM sleep, healthy nutrients, no alcohol consumption and regular physical activities).
- SARS-CoV2 vaccination in the US, especially for the communities of color, namely AA/ Blacks, Hispanics and American Indians for national herd immunity.
- Consistent virtual/digital public health education on SARS-CoV2 transmission and COVID-19 mortality risk factor reduction.

Questions for Discussion

1. Explain how population density in any celebration or event could increase viral transmission such as SARS-CoV2.
2. What measures are required to be in place if the community encourages gathering in any given setting?
3. Describe how a healthy lifestyle could marginalize SARS-CoV2 and any viral spread during Christmas in any population setting.

Notes

1 "SARS-CoV-2 Variants of Concern as of 3 March 2022", https://www.ecdc.europa.eu/en/covid-19/variants-concern. Accessed 9 Mar. 2022.
2 "Tracking Variants – CDPH – CA.gov", https://www.cdph.ca.gov/Programs/CID/DCDC/Pages/COVID-19/COVID-Variants.aspx. Accessed 9 Mar. 2022.

3 "How to Protect Yourself & Others | CDC", https://www.cdc.gov/coronavirus/2019-ncov/prevent-getting-sick/prevention.html. Accessed 9 Mar. 2022.

4 "Viral Load and Contact Heterogeneity Predict SARS-CoV-2 … – eLife". 23 Feb. 2021, https://elifesciences.org/articles/63537. Accessed 9 Mar. 2022.

5 "Molecular Biology of Coronaviruses: Current Knowledge – ScienceDirect". 12 Aug. 2020, https://www.sciencedirect.com/science/article/pii/S2405844020315863. Accessed 9 Mar. 2022.

6 "Understanding Transmission of SARS-CoV-2 in the Ongoing COVID …". 15 Dec. 2021, https://ncceh.ca/documents/evidence-review/understanding-transmission-sars-cov-2-ongoing-covid-19-pandemic. Accessed 9 Mar. 2022.

7 "How Do Viruses Mutate and What it Means for a Vaccine? | Pfizer", https://www.pfizer.com/news/articles/how_do_viruses_mutate_and_what_it_means_for_a_vaccine. Accessed 9 Mar. 2022.

8 "Severe Acute Respiratory Syndrome Coronavirus-2 (SARS-CoV-2)", https://www.ncbi.nlm.nih.gov/pmc/articles/PMC7286265/. Accessed 9 Mar. 2022.

9 "Face Masks Against COVID-19: An Evidence Review – Preprints.org", https://www.preprints.org/manuscript/202004.0203/v1. Accessed 9 Mar. 2022.

10 "COVID-19: Restoring Public Trust During A Global Health Crisis". 22 Feb. 2021, https://olis.oregonlegislature.gov/liz/2021R1/Downloads/PublicTestimonyDocument/8038. Accessed 9 Mar. 2022.

11 "The Path to the Next Normal – McKinsey", https://www.mckinsey.com/~/media/McKinsey/Featured%20Insights/Navigating%20the%20coronavirus%20crisis%20collected%20works/Path-to-the-next-normal-collection.pdf. Accessed 9 Mar. 2022.

12 "Latest Data on COVID-19 Vaccinations by Race/Ethnicity | KFF". 9 Mar. 2022, https://www.kff.org/coronavirus-covid-19/issue-brief/latest-data-on-covid-19-vaccinations-by-race-ethnicity/. Accessed 9 Mar. 2022.

13 "Racial and Ethnic Disparities in the Quality of Health Care – Annual …", https://www.annualreviews.org/doi/10.1146/annurev-publhealth-032315-021439. Accessed 9 Mar. 2022.

14 "Access to COVID-19 Vaccines: Global Approaches in a Global Crisis". 18 Mar. 2021, https://www.oecd.org/coronavirus/policy-responses/access-to-covid-19-vaccines-global-approaches-in-a-global-crisis-c6a18370/. Accessed 9 Mar. 2022

16 SARS-CoV2 (COVID-19) Novel Variants (Delta), Vaccine Cross-Effectiveness and Durability

Vaccine Cross-Reactivity and Community Herd Immunity

The current mRNA vaccine, which had been illustrated to be efficacious, and effective, in human populations – especially the most vulnerable populations and those with the disproportionate burden of COVID-19 mortality namely racial/ethnic minorities in the US and those with chronic conditions/comorbidities who must be vaccinated in a timely manner. Public health institutions in the nation must apply disproportionate universalism in vaccine distribution and administration, implying the subpopulations that are disproportionately affected should be prioritized in this vaccination.[1,2] There are no data currently available to implicate the effectiveness of this mRNA in ensuring antibody cross-reactivity as well as the immune responsiveness with CD4 and CD8 cells with the novel SARS-CoV2 variant.[3] However, where individuals vaccinated with the current mRNA vaccine, exposed to the novel SARS-CoV2 variants, present with clinical manifestations and are hospitalized, thus implying an immunogenicity gap with the current mRNA vaccine, there is a scientific need for cautious optimism in this herd immunity advancement.[4]

Public Health Recommendations and Scientific Community Trajectory

As the scientific communities await the data on the virulence variability (initial SARS-CoV2 versus novel variants) and the current mRNA vaccine durability as well as the anticipated immunogenicity gap with the novel SARS-CoV2 variants,[5] the scientific communities and public health officers must recommend the following guidelines for SARS-CoV2 control and prevention:

- Adherence to the current preventive and control measures for all those who have been vaccinated, namely face mask wearing, social and physical distancing and rigorous hand hygiene.
- Highly coordinated effort for vaccine administration in meeting the current vaccine distribution, which implies the administration of an estimated 33.3% of all the distributed vaccines.
- States, counties and cities must provide resources to the socially disadvantaged populations to access and receive the vaccine for herd immunity in these most vulnerable populations, namely Blacks/AA, Hispanics and American Indians/Alaska Natives.

Since the novel SARS-CoV2 variants are highly transmissible relative to the initial SARS-CoV2, implying exponential case positivity, there is a need for collective adherence to the ongoing preventive and control measures for SARS-CoV2 transmission and infectivity, namely face mask wearing, which protects all, social and physical distancing and rigorous hand hygiene. Therefore, failure to apply these measures, despite the ongoing vaccination progress for herd

DOI: 10.4324/9781003424451-16

immunity, will lead to increased case positivity and excess mortality from this COVID-19 pandemic. Since there are no data on the immunogenic effect of this current mRNA on the current novel variant, there is a probability of an immunogenicity gap, implying SARS-CoV2 novel variants' intensive genomic sequence analysis. With this adherence to scientific data, as it becomes available, efficacious and effective vaccine development will ensure COVID-19 case fatality and mortality marginalization.

With the current scientific data, we need to globally apply these data in a reliable and valid nature for SARS-CoV2 novel variant transmission reduction and COVID-19 case fatality and mortality marginalization.[6] Additionally, since clinical data on COVID-19 complications and comorbidities are not fully understood, and given the potential for chronic disease following recovery and survival from COVID-19, there must be global preventive and control measures across all populations regardless of social status.[7]

Novel SARS-CoV2 Strain Emergence

The mitigation, control and prevention of pathogenic microbes depends on restricted mutation of the viral pathogen, implying less antigenic subtype variabilities. Specifically, the shorter the duration or occurrence of the pathogen in the human population (decreased prevalence) the fewer the variants and antigenic subtypes, indicative of optimal health outcomes.[8,9,10] With SARS-CoV2, given this prolonged period of transmission, there have emerged these mutated strains such as the delta variant.[11] In addressing the transmissibility of this variant, the more communities are vaccinated, the lower the risk of transmission of the delta variant of SARS-CoV2.[12] With the observed increase in delta variant transmission in the US, indicative of international transmission, one recommends global immunization in increasing global herd immunity in handling this pandemic.[13] The WHO requires an instant global health immunization program in engaging with the industrialized nations in the world for global vaccine distribution, especially in nations disproportionately affected by this transmission, namely India and Brazil.[14]

Marginalized Vaccine Uptake and SARS-CoV2 Delta Variant

The current data on the delta variant or strain reflects occurrence in 41 states in the nation as well as hyper-transmissibility, relative to the previous strains of SARS-CoV2 (A/B). As this delta strain has become dominant in the UK, it is highly likely that similar observation of this highly contagious pathogen will be seen here in the US.[15] In effect, given our limited knowledge of antibody cross-reactivity, implying enhanced immunogenicity, if already vaccinated individuals are exposed to the new variants, SARS-CoV2 delta, there should be a substantial immune response (immunoglobulins, active T-cells and NK-cells integration) in protecting against infectivity regardless of exposure.[16] With this observation, despite our limited knowledge of this pathogen as an extra respiratory and pulmonary pathogenic microbe, we firmly recommend all Americans deemed eligible for this immunization to be vaccinated. Second, we recommend the distribution and allocation of the current vaccines, which does not involve the most recent delta variant (mRNA or toxoid), to the underdeveloped and developing countries for global herd immunity and pandemic mitigation, in returning the world to the pre–SARS-CoV2 health survivability and stability.[17]

Delta Variant Spread Marginalization: Epigenomic Public Health Dimensions

As public health inclines to the implication of the environment in disease process, prognosis, mortality and survival, and the community approach to disease control and prevention, we must embrace the notion of epigenomic public health both in the current and future pandemic mitigation and stabilization.[18] Specifically, epigenomic public health reflects the gene and environment interaction in the societal consideration of how social, psychosocial, exogenous, endogenous, physical, chemical and economic environment as social gradient impacts on epigenomic modulations, adversely impacting transcriptomes resulting in inverse gene expression and adverse cellular functionality, due to dysfunctionality in gene expression and protein synthesis at the subpopulation level.[19] Clearly, environmental variabilities reflect subpopulation differentials in treatment response as reflected in drug receptors and tissue remodeling post surgically, implying an equitable environment in addressing subpopulation variances in vaccine response, adverse vaccine effects and treatment during pandemics.[20]

Questions for Discussion

1. Explain vaccine cross-reactivity and implication in community herd immunity enhancement.
2. With respect to new SARS-CoV2 strain or variants, what are the public health recommendations in controlling the spread of this pathogenic microbe?
3. Regarding SARS-CoV2 novel variant, explain the preventive measures including ongoing vaccination in novel SARS-CoV2 community transmission.
4. Describe SARS-CoV2 delta variant and examine the antigen variability between the initial SARS-CoV2 and the delta variant.
5. Provide a brief description of epigenomic public health and the application of this novel dimension of public health in SARS-CoV2 transmissibility reduction.
6. Does the current SARS-CoV2 mRNA vaccine provide some protection among the vaccinated individuals compared to the un-vaccinated?
7. Since the world community reflects a global village, examine the WHO initiative in addressing the current SARS-CoV2 variant.

Notes

1 "NEUROLOGICAL DISORDERS – WHO | World Health Organization", https://www.who.int/mental_health/neurology/neurological_disorders_report_web.pdf. Accessed 9 Mar. 2022.
2 "Insights to SARS-CoV-2 Life Cycle, Pathophysiology, and Rationalized …". 12 Jan. 2021, https://jbiomedsci.biomedcentral.com/articles/10.1186/s12929-020-00703-5. Accessed 9 Mar. 2022.
3 "Two Different Antibody-Dependent Enhancement (ADE) Risks for …". 24 Feb. 2021, https://www.frontiersin.org/articles/10.3389/fimmu.2021.640093/full. Accessed 9 Mar. 2022.
4 "Development of SARS-CoV-2 Vaccines: Challenges, Risks, and the …", https://www.ncbi.nlm.nih.gov/pmc/articles/PMC7754925/. Accessed 9 Mar. 2022.
5 "Risk of SARS-CoV-2 Transmission from Newly … – ECDC". 29 Mar. 2021, https://www.ecdc.europa.eu/sites/default/files/documents/Risk-of-transmission-and-reinfection-of-SARS-CoV-2-following-vaccination.pdf. Accessed 9 Mar. 2022.
6 "Summary of Guidance for Public Health Strategies to Address High …". 11 Dec. 2020, https://www.cdc.gov/mmwr/volumes/69/wr/mm6949e2.htm. Accessed 9 Mar. 2022.
7 "COVID-19 (Novel Coronavirus) – DynaMed", https://www.dynamed.com/condition/covid-19-novel-coronavirus. Accessed 9 Mar. 2022.
8 "Immunization in the United States: Recommendations, Barriers, and …", https://www.ncbi.nlm.nih.gov/pmc/articles/PMC4927017/. Accessed 9 Mar. 2022.
9 "The Effects of Virus Variants on COVID-19 Vaccines – WHO | World …". 1 Mar. 2021, https://www.who.int/news-room/feature-stories/detail/the-effects-of-virus-variants-on-covid-19-vaccines. Accessed 9 Mar. 2022.
10 "COVID Variants: What You Should Know | Johns Hopkins Medicine". 14 Jan. 2022, https://www.hopkinsmedicine.org/health/conditions-and-diseases/coronavirus/a-new-strain-of-coronavirus-what-you-should-know. Accessed 9 Mar. 2022.
11 "Tracking SARS-CoV-2 Variants – WHO | World Health Organization", https://www.who.int/en/activities/tracking-SARS-CoV-2-variants/. Accessed 9 Mar. 2022.

12 "How do Vaccinated People Spread Delta? What the Science Says". 12 Aug. 2021, https://www.nature.com/articles/d41586-021-02187-1. Accessed 9 Mar. 2022.
13 "COVID-19: Epidemiology, Virology, and Prevention – UpToDate". 1 Mar. 2022, https://www.uptodate.com/contents/covid-19-epidemiology-virology-and-prevention. Accessed 9 Mar. 2022.
14 "National Strategy for the COVID-19 Response and Pandemic". 21 Jan. 2021, https://www.whitehouse.gov/wp-content/uploads/2021/01/National-Strategy-for-the-COVID-19-Response-and-Pandemic-Preparedness.pdf. Accessed 9 Mar. 2022.
15 "SARS-CoV-2 Delta Variant – Wikipedia", https://en.wikipedia.org/wiki/SARS-CoV-2_Delta_variant. Accessed 9 Mar. 2022.
16 "Two Doses of SARS-CoV-2 Vaccination Induce Robust Immune ...". 17 Aug. 2021, https://www.nature.com/articles/s41467-021-25167-5. Accessed 9 Mar. 2022.
17 "Impact of Vaccines; Health, Economic and Social Perspectives". 14 Jul. 2020, https://www.frontiersin.org/articles/10.3389/fmicb.2020.01526/full. Accessed 9 Mar. 2022.
18 "Health Inequalities and Infectious Disease Epidemics: A Challenge ...", https://www.ncbi.nlm.nih.gov/pmc/articles/PMC4170985/. Accessed 9 Mar. 2022.
19 "Social Epigenetics and Equality of Opportunity – NCBI". 15 Jul. 2013, https://www.ncbi.nlm.nih.gov/pmc/articles/PMC3712403/. Accessed 9 Mar. 2022.
20 "Statement for Healthcare Professionals: How COVID-19 Vaccines ...", https://www.who.int/news/item/11-06-2021-statement-for-healthcare-professionals-how-covid-19-vaccines-are-regulated-for-safety-and-effectiveness. Accessed 9 Mar. 2022.

17 SARS-CoV2 (COVID-19) Disproportionate Burden

Hypertension and Mental Health among US Racial/Ethnic Minorities – Blacks/African Americans (AA)

Health Disparities, Comorbidities and SARS-CoV2 Transmissibility

Historically, and till date, Blacks/ AA have experienced the disproportionate burden of morbidity and mortality in the US. As reflected by Rev. Martin Luther King, of all forms of social injustice, the most shocking and staggering is that of health disparities.[1] This perception and observation was accurate then and is still accurate today. The question remains, what is the cause or causes of morbidity and mortality racial variance, and how could we as a nation transform health equity?[2]

Whereas medicine as a science had implicated genetic variability in disease development and outcomes such as cystic fibrosis and sickle cell anemia/disease, there are several clinical conditions, such as hypertension (HTN), asthma, cardiomyopathies, angina pectoris, Type II diabetes, COPD, autoimmune disorders, malignant neoplasm, and cerebrovascular accident[3] that are driven by aberrant epigenomic modulations, implying impaired gene and environment interaction. Simply, it is not genetic variability comparing Blacks/AA and their White counterparts that predispose the communities of color to the disproportionate burden of morbidity and mortality in COVID-19, given the genomic similarities (<0.05% of DNA sequencing), but the gene and environment interaction in SARS-CoV2 transmission/seropositivity and COVID-19 disease development, prognosis, outcome, survival and mortality.[4]

With the ongoing racial variances or disparities in eHTN outcomes and the implication of this clinical condition in SARS-CoV2 transmission, infectivity and COVID-19 severity as well as complications and mortality, [5] there is an urgent need to transform health equity in this nation, state and local government through the provision of equitable resources to the communities of color namely Blacks/AA, Hispanics/Latino and American Indians/Alaska Natives.[6] This initiative reflects the public health concept of disproportionate universalism, implying that equitable resources be allocated to the populations requiring substantial health needs.[7] The disproportionate burden of SARS-CoV2 transmission, case fatality and mortality among populations with comorbidities namely AA/Blacks is explained by social injustice and health inequity, implying unjust and unfair allocation of economic, social and environmental resources related to human health.[8]

SARS-CoV2 and COVID-19: Black/African Americans (AA) Transmission and Mortality Experience

The SARS-CoV2 transmission and COVID-19 case fatality, survival and mortality has disproportionately affected communities of color, especially Blacks/AA and Hispanics.[9] This disproportionate burden is due to social and health inequity driven by social injustice which marginalizes value healthcare and optimal preventive health services, including timely cancer screening, as reflected in inadequate health insurance coverage that adversely impacts care

DOI: 10.4324/9781003424451-17

access and utilization.[10] In addressing this health and healthcare destabilization among Blacks/ AA in the nation, there is a need for policy development, implementation and evaluation that allows for appropriate care utilization regardless of insurance coverage, since human health is a primary and not secondary value and should not be dependent on the type of insurance coverage. The observed health destabilization of Blacks/AA in COVID-19 is clearly attributable to health inequity that renders the most vulnerable populations to impaired health outcomes in any condition – including the COVID-19 pandemic.[11]

Blacks/AA living in high population density neighborhoods are more likely to be exposed to pathogenic microbes including SARS-CoV2 and the novel variants of SARS-CoV2. Second, Blacks/AA are more predisposed to COVID-19 complications, poor prognosis and mortality as well as survival disadvantage due to primary HTN as a pre-existing condition, given SARS-CoV-2 receptor affinity with patients placed on ACE inhibitor medications.[12] The prevalence of primary HTN, and other cardiovascular disorders such as cerebrovascular accident (stroke), is higher among Blacks/AA relative to their White counterparts, which explains. in part. the excess mortality and survival disadvantage of Blacks/AA with COVID-19.[13]

Blacks/AA and Essential/Primary Hypertension (HTN) in COVID-19 Pandemic

Essential or primary HTN hypertension, despite its genomic implication in predisposition, epigenomic modulations which are transgenerational but reversible, explains the highest prevalence of this condition among Blacks/AA in the US. Multifactorial etiology explains this excess prevalence among Blacks/AA namely physical, psychological, endogenous, exogenous and social environment.[14] The interaction of this environment with HTN genes associated with HTN biomarkers such as Angiotensin Converting Enzyme (ACE) that converts Angiotensin (I) to A-II, a potent vasoconstrictor, enhancing peripheral resistance and vasoconstriction, thus induced an obstacle to the flow of blood. In addition, exposure to stress, subordination, [15] discrimination and racism provokes the sympathetic response, thus increasing the elaboration of norepinephrine and epinephrine, leading to vasoconstriction and essential HTN. Basically, HTN is explained by cardiac output (CO) and peripheral resistance (PR) which in combination reflects volume loading and depletion as implicated in the heart rate, stroke volumes and stenosis, inducing systolic and diastolic blood pressure elevation.[16]

Blacks/AA with essential HTN require vaccination, given the current SARS-CoV2 variants in the US as well as the observed excess case fatality and mortality in this population relative to their White counterparts.[17] This recommendation validates the public health notion of disproportionate universalism that requires disproportionate benefit for populations with the disproportionate burden of the disease such as Blacks/AA with COVID-19.[18] Additionally, with the required vaccine and the current SARS-CoV2 variants, there is a need for all vaccinated populations to adhere to face mask wearing, social distancing and rigorous hand hygiene, since an estimated 5% of those who have been vaccinated may become re-infected, especially given the novel SARS-CoV2 variants, implying the potential for decreased antibody protection from the South African, and Brazililian SARS-CoV2 variants.[19]

Mental/Behavioral Dysfunction among Blacks/AA and Therapeutics Recommendation in COVID-19 Pandemic

The epigenomic modulations of the central nervous system play a substantial role in mental illness, given cortisol response to socially isolated environments, predisposing to major depressive episodes. Blacks/AA have the highest prevalence of psychological and mental disorders in the US which is attributable to racial discrimination, socioeconomic deprivation, systemic racism, police brutality, and social injustice/inequity. With the Black History Month, we encourage the Black/AA population to apply integrative care such as medication, counseling and spirituality in addressing this condition, thus lowering the prevalence of mental illness and improving the health and educational achievement among Blacks/AA in the US.[20]

With the COVID-19 pandemic and the historical reality of the disproportionate burden of pandemics among Blacks/AA in the nation, the Black History Month remains an agenda for all communities of color, especially Blacks/AA, to reflect on how the environment interacts with the biologic system, mainly genes, and predispose humanity to adverse health conditions.[21] While the aberrant epigenomic modulations are more common among Blacks/AA relative to Whites in the nation, these changes despite being transgenerational are reversible, implying our collective initiative as Blacks/AA to modify these environments (social, psychological, socioeconomic, physical, etc.,) through policies aimed at restoring social equity, social justice and health equity. Therefore, the inability to formulate, implement and evaluate these policies for intervention mapping in transforming health equity, will continue to subject Blacks/AA in the nation to the disproportionate burden of morbidity and mortality.[22]

Questions for Discussion

1. What is the epigenomic mechanistic process and aberrant epigenomic modulation in morbidity, prognosis and survival?
2. Explain how aberrant epigenomic modulations increase hypertension in some subpopulations, and the implication of this comorbidity in SARS-CoV2 transmission and COVID-19 mortality.
3. Examine health disparities in the US and the implication of racial/ethnic disparities in the disproportionate burden of ICU admissions and poor prognosis among COVID-19 patients.
4. Review the article by Holmes, L Jr on aberrant epigenomic modulation of the hypertension gene – https://pubmed.ncbi.nlm.nih.gov/31689998/. Explain the implication of conserved transcriptional response to adversity (CTRA) gene in HTN as well as SARS-CoV2.

Notes

1 "The State of Health Disparities in the United States – NCBI", https://www.ncbi.nlm.nih.gov/books/NBK425844/. Accessed 9 Mar. 2022.
2 "Health Disparity – An Overview | ScienceDirect Topics", https://www.sciencedirect.com/topics/biochemistry-genetics-and-molecular-biology/health-disparity. Accessed 9 Mar. 2022.
3 "Recommendations and Guidelines for Preoperative Evaluation", https://www.unmc.edu/media/anesthesia/Anesthesia%20Guide.pdf. Accessed 9 Mar. 2022.
4 "Environment and Gene Association With Obesity and Their Impact …". 28 Aug. 2020, https://www.frontiersin.org/articles/565326. Accessed 9 Mar. 2022.
5 "Racial and Ethnic Differences in Presentation and Outcomes for …". 17 Nov. 2020, https://www.ahajournals.org/doi/10.1161/CIRCULATIONAHA.120.052278. Accessed 9 Mar. 2022.
6 "Embed Racial Justice and Advance Health Equity – American …". 6 May. 2021, https://www.ama-assn.org/system/files/2021–05/ama-equity-strategic-plan.pdf. Accessed 9 Mar. 2022.
7 "A Conceptual Framework For Action on the Social Determinants …", https://www.who.int/sdhconference/resources/ConceptualframeworkforactiononSDH_eng.pdf. Accessed 9 Mar. 2022.
8 "Visualizing COVID-19 Mortality Rates and African-American … - NCBI". 9 Feb. 2021, https://www.ncbi.nlm.nih.gov/pmc/articles/PMC7872308/. Accessed 9 Mar. 2022.
9 "Health Equity Considerations and Racial and Ethnic Minority Groups", https://www.cdc.gov/coronavirus/2019-ncov/community/health-equity/race-ethnicity.html. Accessed 9 Mar. 2022.
10 "Understanding and Addressing Social Determinants to Advance …", https://acsjournals.onlinelibrary.wiley.com/doi/full/10.3322/caac.21586. Accessed 9 Mar. 2022.

11 "Health Equity Considerations and Racial and Ethnic Minority Groups", https://www.cdc.gov/coronavirus/2019-ncov/community/health-equity/race-ethnicity.html. Accessed 9 Mar. 2022.

12 "Coronavirus Disease 2019 (COVID-19) – Medscape Reference", https://emedicine.medscape.com/article/2500114-overview. Accessed 9 Mar. 2022.

13 "Belated Black History Month Reflection: SARS-Cov2 (COVID-19 …". 7 Mar. 2021, https://www.linkedin.com/pulse/belated-black-history-month-reflection-sars-cov2-larry-. Accessed 9 Mar. 2022.

14 "Obesity-Related Hypertension: Possible Pathophysiological …", https://joe.bioscientifica.com/downloadpdf/journals/joe/223/3/R63.xml. Accessed 9 Mar. 2022.

15 "ACE Inhibitor – Wikipedia", https://en.wikipedia.org/wiki/ACE_inhibitor. Accessed 9 Mar. 2022.

16 "Cardiac and Vascular Pathophysiology in Hypertension – NCBI", https://www.ncbi.nlm.nih.gov/pmc/articles/PMC1767863/. Accessed 9 Mar. 2022.

17 "Pandemics Throughout History | Microbiology – Frontiers". 15 Jan. 2021, https://www.frontiersin.org/articles/10.3389/fmicb.2020.631736/full. Accessed 9 Mar. 2022.

18 "Disparities in Health and Health Care: 5 Key Questions and Answers". 11 May. 2021, https://www.kff.org/racial-equity-and-health-policy/issue-brief/disparities-in-health-and-health-care-5-key-question-and-answers/. Accessed 9 Mar. 2022.

19 "COVID-19 Vaccination and Testing; Emergency Temporary Standard". 5 Nov. 2021, https://www.federalregister.gov/documents/2021/11/05/2021–23643/covid-19-vaccination-and-testing-emergency-temporary-standard. Accessed 9 Mar. 2022.

20 "Black/African American | SAMHSA", https://www.samhsa.gov/behavioral-health-equity/black-african-american. Accessed 9 Mar. 2022.

21 "Impact of Social Determinants of Health on the Emerging COVID-19 …". 21 Jul. 2020, https://www.frontiersin.org/articles/10.3389/fpubh.2020.00406/full. Accessed 9 Mar. 2022.

22 "Combined Frequency-amplitude Nonlinear Modulation – arXiv", https://arxiv.org/pdf/0902.4901. Accessed 9 Mar. 2022.

18 SARS-CoV2 Delta Variant (B.1.617.2) Transmissibility, Subpopulations Case-Positivity, Case Fatality and Mortality

Background and Significance

The delta variant is clearly a more contagious SARS-CoV2 strains compared to the alpha and beta strains, requiring immediate and rapid vaccination of all vaccine-eligible Americans and the global population.[1,2] Therefore, the departure from this recommendation reflects the emergence of a new variant ("delta-2") due to marginalized community herd immunity and current delta exponential spread among the unvaccinated individuals, leading to increased case fatality and mortality in this subpopulation with vaccine hesitancy.[3,4,5] These data-driven observations are suggestive of immediate vaccination of all vaccine-eligible Americans for herd immunity attainment, as well as mask wearing, social and physical distancing and rigorous hand hygiene, until community herd immunity is achieved with an estimated 70–85% of the US population vaccinated.[6,7]

The current surge in COVID-19 is due primarily to the SARS-CoV2 mutant; termed the delta variant, which had been observed with 1,000 times viral load relative to the early SARS-Cov2 strains 19A – alpha (B.1.1.7) and 19B (B.1.351). Available epidemiologic and clinical data observed exponential transmissibility, case fatality, hospitalization, and replication rate, ICU admission and mortality in the current delta variant, termed a variant of concern (VOC). Whereas immunization based on the current viral strains namely 19A/20A do not offer 100% immuno-potentiation as a result of antibody cross-reactivity,[8] the current SARS-Cov2 vaccines (Pfizer, Moderna, and to some extent Johnson & Johnson) had been observed with substantial antibody reactivity with respect to the delta variant.

With the limited knowledge of the current vaccine efficacy and effectiveness based on SARS-CoV2 alpha and beta strains, and its cross-protectivity for the delta variant, there is an urgent and immediate need for all individuals, clinically termed vaccine-eligible, to be immunized for community herd immunity attainment and return to the pre-COVID-19 pandemic era.[9] Therefore, failure to apply this scientific recommendation on translational immuno-epidemiologic perspective, will result in ample opportunity for delta variant mutation, that may lead to another novel variant (delta-2) which certainly will be more contagious than the current delta variant, with the adverse outcomes being increased hospitalization, poor prognosis, complications and excess mortality. Whereas misinformation and fear tend to drive the current vaccine hesitancy in the US, and the unfortunate pediatric mortality with the delta variant as well as noncompliance and adherence to public health viral/pathogenic microbe control and preventive measures,[10] this translational immuno-epidemiologic perspective attempts to present a reliable and meaningful data on: (a) delta variant genomics and transmissibility, (b) subpopulation variances in delta variant case positivity, (c) case-fatality and mortality, as well as a recommendation for the US population to return to the pre–COVID-19 pandemic era.

DOI: 10.4324/9781003424451-18

Materials and Methods

A qualitative systematic review and Qualitative Evidence Synthesis (QES) was used to assess the published literature on SARS-CoV2 variants as mutants. This approach involved the application of a search engine and identification of search terms in the relevant literature, and the application of manuscripts' quality criteria in the utilization of such findings in the QES.

Results

A qualitative systematic review was applied in assessing published literature on SARS-CoV2 genomics with respect to mutation and strains, US case positivity, clinical manifestations (disease severity), hospitalization and mortality, comparing initial variants (alpha and beta) with the current variant, delta. Available data indicate variabilities in the S gene mutation of the alpha, beta and delta strains, with hyper-mutation or several mutations associated with delta variant relative to the initial strains, which reflects higher vulnerability, replication and exponential transmissibility.[4] The QES reflects synopsis in the reviewed literature as observed below, namely the delta variant genomics and spread, subpopulation variability in the delta variant transmissibility, vaccine hesitancy, case fatality and mortality.

Delta Variant (B.1.617.2) Genomics and Transmissibility

The first detected case of B.1.617.2, a SARS-CoV2 lineage, was in India during December 2020. However, today this strain is observed in all states in the US, accounting for more than 83% of all new cases of COVID-19 as SARS-CoV2 positivity.[11] Reliable epidemiologic data observed greater than 60% increased risk of transmission (absolute incidence difference) of this

Table 18.1 SARS-CoV2 Variants Genomic Characterization

Variable/Viral Particles	Alpha Variant	Beta Variant	Delta Variant
Mutagenic Code	B.1.1.7	B.1.351	B.617.2
Spike (S) protein (D614, G614) – estimated 1255 (aa) transmembrane protein facilitates viral attachment and host cell penetration.	↑ACE2, Antibodies or B-cells alteration, immune escape, ineffective monoclonal antibodies	↑ACE2, Antibodies or B-cells alteration, immune escape, ineffective monoclonal antibodies	↑↑↑ACE2, Antibodies or B-cells alteration, immune escape, hyper ineffective monoclonal antibodies
Geographic variance	Wuhan, China	USA, Europe, South Africa, Africa	India, USA, Europe, South America
Host factor	ACE2, TMPRSS2, HLA, CD147, MIF, IFNG, IL6	ACE2, TMPRSS2, HLA, CD147, MIF, IFNG, IL6	ACE2, TMPRSS2, HLA, CD147, MIF, IFNG, IL6

Notes and abbreviations: The S protein (D614G), the most predominant, significantly increases SARS-CoV2 transmission the US and Europe. The host inert and adaptive immune system besides genetic variants modulate susceptibility, disease severity, symptoms manifestation, and immune responsiveness against SARS-CoV2. A single AA mutation within spike glycoprotein alters Angiotensin Converting Enzyme (ACE II) binding as well as B-cell epitopes in enhancing immune escape and ineffective monoclonal antibodies response to SARS-CoV2. Overall, non-structural and accessory proteins can enhance antibody resistance to antivirals, T-cell epitopes alteration and cell mediated immune responsiveness impairment.

strain relative to the alpha variant, first observed in England during the early months of 2020. The delta variant of the COVID-19 pathogenic microbe has been observed with 1,000 times viral load, relative to alpha and beta variants.[12] The delta variant as a VOC reflects an exponential transmission, implying nine transmissibility relative to two to three transmissions with alpha and delta variants as original variant following contact with an infected individual. The delta variant data in July are indicative of exponential spread, as reflected in 530% daily incident cases, 160% hospitalization and 43% daily mortality.

The SARS-CoV2 B.1.617.2 is identified with the S gene mutation, including variants or mutations in the receptor binding domain (RBD), which is located close to the furin cleavage site as well as mutations in the vulnerable region of the N-terminal domain in antibody or immunoglobulin, termed antigenic supersite.[13] This RBD is the part or portion of the spike (S) protein that binds to human animal ACE2 receptors, leading to viral replication in the host. The B.1.617.2 is associated with three RBD mutations, namely lysine to asparagine, leucine to arginine, and threonine to lysine.[14] These mutations are also associated with beta variants (lysine to asparagine), and results in increased RBD-ACE2 binding affinity, resulting in immuno-downregulation, enabling immune escape. Regarding the spike protein, it comprises a receptor binding subunit (S1) and fusion subunit (S2), resulting in cleavage membrane fusion mediation and viral replication as well as infectivity. Within the cleavage site, delta is characterized by proline to arginine substitution which is also observed in the alpha variant.[15] Due to these mutations, more S proteins are primed to access human cells and enhance replication, hence infectivity. With the ongoing data, the original strain was associated with <10% S protein priming, an estimated 50% in the alpha variant, while >75% was associated with respect to priming in the delta variant. With respect to other initial variants, the delta variant had been observed with the

Table 18.2 SARS-CoV2 Variants and Immunogenicity

Variable/Viral Particles	Alpha Variant	Beta Variant	Delta Variant
Antibodies	Moderate immunoglobulin response	Moderate immunoglobulin response	Low immunoglobulin response
Unvaccinated – exposure to SARS-CoV2	Moderately contagious	Moderately contagious	Highly contagious – 1,000 times viral load relative to alpha and beta variant
Vaccinated – individual uptake	Low transmissibility opportunity	Low transmissibility opportunity	High transmissibility opportunity
Vaccinated – organ transplant	Increased antibodies, T-cells and NKC integration	Increased antibodies, T-cells and NKC integration	Increased antibodies, T-cells and NKC integration
Vaccinated – immunosuppressive agent	Increased immune response – antibodies with boaster shots	Increased immune response – antibodies with boaster shots	Increased immune response – antibodies with boaster shots

Notes: Due to antibody variability with these variants, vaccination result in immunopotentiation. Individual vaccinated have increased immune protection requiring increasing vaccines for herd immunity. With the current data, a booster shot is required among immunosuppressed individuals and those with organ transplants. Natural immunity from infected individuals although more protective as generated from the viral pathogen, from the infected individuals, vaccine uptake is required in enhancing further immunopotentiation.

N-terminal domain region of the S protein, termed NTD-antigenic supersites, which is vulnerable to antibody recognition and attack/destruction.

Subpopulation Variances in Delta Variant Case Positivity: Vaccine Hesitancy

The delta variant has currently been observed with increased seropositivity among children, adolescents and young adults. The observed subpopulation seropositivity and transmissibility increase or excess transmission and infectivity is due, in greater part, to decreased or marginalized SARS-CoV2 immunization.[16] Specifically, as observed in the history of pathogenic microbes, as the herd immunity decreases due to the inability or unwillingness (vaccine hesitancy) of the human society to be immunized, the greater the viral mutation and increasing strains and variants, implying decreased host immune responsiveness and defense, resulting in increasing contagiousness/transmissibility, clinical manifestations, complications and survival disadvantage. Immunologic observation implicates exponential spread of any pathogenic microbe to increase viral mutation.[17] Specifically, the less populations remain "unimmunized", implying unvaccinated individuals in a given specific population (lower herd immunity), the higher the viral transmissibility. Available and reliable data indicates 70–85% of the immunized population with herd immunity. However, in the US, an estimated 49.9% (349 million administered vaccines) are currently vaccinated, implying lack of herd immunity in COVID-19.

The current data (July/August, 2021) on SARS-CoV2 transmission in the US have implicated Louisiana, Texas, Florida, Arkansas and Alabama with the lowest vaccination rates relative to other states, which explains the increasing delta variant case positivity, increased hospitalization, limited ICU space and increased mortality in COVID-19 in these states.[18] A careful assessment of SARS-CoV2 strains, alpha, beta and delta with respect to the S gene mutation, explains the protective effect of the current vaccine (Moderna, Pfizer, Johnson & Johnson) on individuals exposed to the delta variant after vaccination. Simply the S gene mutation observed in delta incorporates the mutation aspect of the alpha and beta variant. Since the current variant is based on S gene mutations with alpha and beta strains, there is a potential for 66.6% to 75% of the immune responsiveness (immunogenicity) among individuals exposed to the delta variant, implying low infectivity among vaccinated individuals with exponential spread, as nine to ten times as likely for transmission, relative to two to three times with alpha and beta variants. Among the vaccinated individuals in the US, an estimated 99.9% have not been hospitalized following exposure to delta variant, while >88% of unvaccinated individuals with delta variant case positivity have been observed with hospitalization and severe clinical manifestations.[19]

Children and young adults, relative to the elderly, are observed with high delta variant exponential transmission, which is explained by low immunization in this subpopulation. The misinformation from social media on the effectiveness and risk, including infertility, tends to enhance vaccine hesitancy among adolescents and young adults as well as older adults. While social media is the platform for information dissemination today, it is, however, very unfortunate that such information requires data verification prior to application in decision making pertaining to human health, a primary value.[20]

Regarding current information on the COVID-19 vaccine, information reliability requires the assessment of the available data on mechanism of action, immune responsiveness, effectiveness, safety and adverse effects from reliable data sources despite the incompleteness of this information, since no scientific data are completely certain, sufficient and consistent, with all scientific findings driven by some uncertainty, random error quantification.[21] These reliable data for decision making regarding vaccination are available at the US Center for Disease Control and Prevention (CDC), American Public Health Association, Royal Society of Medicine, American Medical Association, American College of Epidemiology, etc.

COVID-19 Spike (Delta Variant), Case-Fatality and Mortality

Available epidemiologic data on weekly transmission in June, July and August 2020, in states with lowest vaccination rates in the US, reflects the COVID-19 spike, indicative of exponential spread of the delta variant in these specific populations. The July weekly spread, with an estimated case positivity of 93,996, indicates a 48% increase from the previous week, while mortality data observed 426 deaths of the weekly average and 41% increased mortality when proportionally compared to the previous week (364 deaths, 38% increased mortality compared with the previous week).[22] Since 99.9% of vaccinated individuals had no breakthrough case, implying <0.1% hospitalization or mortality associated with the delta variant, the understanding of this transmission and replication allows for decision making in vaccine uptake among all vaccine-eligible Americans. Specifically based on the observation of the nasal colonization of the delta variant, 1,000 times viral load relative to alpha and beta variant, there remains exponential replication and transmissibility.[23]

The opportunity for viral exponential spread implies viral mutation, and with a constellation of a mutation, may result in a more contagious variant compared to the delta strain. Since an estimated 93 million of eligible Americans remain unvaccinated, there will be a compromised community herd immunity, implying increasing delta variant spread among this vulnerable population, with the opportunity for a novel variant as a result of increasing mutation due to delta variant "freedom and liberty" driven by vaccine hesitancy.[24]

Evidence-Driven Recommendations

The risk and benefit analysis is indicative of the recommendation of the current COVID-19 vaccine for all vaccine-eligible Americans. Historical and current data on vaccine efficacy and effectiveness does not imply 100% efficacy and effectiveness, since there are no vaccines observed in human history without adverse effects. Specifically, unvaccinated individuals, especially adolescents and young/older adults, have severe respiratory conditions and compromised oxygenation as clinical/pathologic manifestations and excess mortality, given delta variant transmission and infectivity relative to alpha and beta variants. The current data requires urgent/rapid vaccination of the US population in obtaining an estimated 70–75% immunization proportion for herd immunity,[25] thus mitigating delta variant mutation and exponential spread as well as highly contagious strain based on hyper-mutation of the novel variant (delta 2).

With the available data on translational immuno-epidemiologic perspective of the delta variant, this observation recommends:

(a) Urgent and immediate requirement of vaccination among all vaccine-eligible Americans to be vaccinated.
(b) Face mask wearing in close environments as well as in public environments, especially without knowledge of those who are vaccinated or not, as well as in subpopulations with a low vaccination rate or proportion, namely Louisiana, Florida, Texas, Alabama, Arkansas.

(c) Physical and social distancing due to the exponential replication and transmission of this delta variant relative to alpha and beta strain.
(d) Rigorous hand hygiene implying hand cleaning with disinfectant, soap and water.

Questions for Discussion

1. What are the objective/s and research question/s in this QES?
2. Describe the aim of this study and the epidemiologic design utilized in this scientific evidence discovery on SARS-CoV2 variants genomic characterization and immunogenicity.
3. What are the main findings in this study?
4. Examine the study limitations and provide suggestions for study improvement.

Notes

1 "The Role of Vaccines in Preventing Bacterial Antimicrobial Resistance". 1 Jan. 2018, https://www.nature.com/articles/nm.4465. Accessed 9 Mar. 2022.
2 "Use of COVID-19 Vaccines After Reports of Adverse Events Among …". 13 Aug. 2021, https://www.cdc.gov/mmwr/volumes/70/wr/mm7032e4.htm. Accessed 9 Mar. 2022.
3 "Science Brief: COVID-19 Vaccines and Vaccination – NCBI", https://www.ncbi.nlm.nih.gov/books/NBK570435/ . Accessed 10 Mar. 2022.
4 "Emergence of SARS-CoV-2 B.1.1.7 Lineage – Centers for Disease …". 22 Jan. 2021, https://www.cdc.gov/mmwr/volumes/70/wr/mm7003e2.htm. Accessed 10 Mar. 2022.
5 "Vaccinated and Unvaccinated Individuals have Similar Viral Loads". 31 Jul. 2021, https://www.medrxiv.org/content/10.1101/2021.07.31.21261387v1. Accessed 10 Mar. 2022.
6 "COVID-19: Epidemiology, Virology, and Prevention – UpToDate". 1 Mar. 2022, https://www.uptodate.com/contents/covid-19-epidemiology-virology-and-prevention. Accessed 10 Mar. 2022.
7 "Investigating the Links Between Vaccination Against COVID-19 and …". 21 Jul. 2021, https://www.frontiersin.org/articles/10.3389/fpubh.2021.702699/full. Accessed 10 Mar. 2022.
8 "COVID-19 Variants | Washington State Department of Health", https://doh.wa.gov/emergencies/covid-19/variants. Accessed 10 Mar. 2022.
9 "Rethinking Herd Immunity and the Covid-19 Response End Game". 13 Sep. 2021, https://publichealth.jhu.edu/2021/what-is-herd-immunity-and-how-can-we-achieve-it-with-covid-19. Accessed 10 Mar. 2022.
10 "COVID-19 and Vaccine Hesitancy: A Longitudinal Study – PLOS". 16 Apr. 2021, https://journals.plos.org/plosone/article?id=10.1371/journal.pone.0250123. Accessed 10 Mar. 2022.
11 "Coronavirus Disease 2019 (COVID-19) Daily Research Briefs", https://www.aafp.org/journals/afp/content/covid-briefs.html. Accessed 10 Mar. 2022.
12 Emergence of SARS-CoV-2 B.1.1.7 Lineage – Centers for Disease …". 22 Jan. 2021, https://www.cdc.gov/mmwr/volumes/70/wr/mm7003e2.htm. Accessed 10 Mar. 2022.
13 "Reduced Sensitivity of SARS-CoV-2 Variant Delta to Antibody …". 8 Jul. 2021, https://www.nature.com/articles/s41586-021-03777-9. Accessed 10 Mar. 2022.
14 "Emerging SARS-CoV-2 Variants of Concern and Potential …". 12 Jul. 2021, https://ccforum.biomedcentral.com/articles/10.1186/s13054-021-03662-x. Accessed 10 Mar. 2022.
15 "How Ominous Is the Omicron Variant (B.1.1.529)? – American …". 16 Dec. 2021, https://asm.org/Articles/2021/December/How-Ominous-is-the-Omicron-Variant-B-1-1-529. Accessed 10 Mar. 2022.
16 "SARS-CoV-2 Vaccines Based on the Spike Glycoprotein … – Frontiers". 12 Jul. 2021, https://www.frontiersin.org/articles/10.3389/fimmu.2021.701501/full. Accessed 10 Mar. 2022.
17 "Vaccination-Induced Herd Immunity: Successes and Challenges". 24 May. 2018, https://www.ncbi.nlm.nih.gov/pmc/articles/PMC6433118/. Accessed 10 Mar. 2022.
18 "COVID-19: TCTMD's Dispatch for March 9 | tctmd.com", https://www.tctmd.com/news/COVID19-daily-dispatch. Accessed 10 Mar. 2022.
19 "Emerging SARS-CoV-2 Variants: A Review of Its Mutations … – NCBI". 18 Oct. 2021, https://www.ncbi.nlm.nih.gov/pmc/articles/PMC8537675/. Accessed 10 Mar. 2022.

20 "Messages from the COVID-19 Response Task Force", https://education.aaaai.org/resources-for-a-i-clinicians/task-force-messages_COVID-19. Accessed 10 Mar. 2022.
21 "Statement for Healthcare Professionals: How COVID-19 Vaccines …". 11 Jun. 2021, https://www.who.int/news/item/11–06–2021-statement-for-healthcare-professionals-how-covid-19-vaccines-are-regulated-for-safety-and-effectiveness. Accessed 10 Mar. 2022.
22 "Rapid Increase in Circulation of the SARS-CoV-2 B.1.617.2 (Delta …". 13 Aug. 2021, https://www.cdc.gov/mmwr/volumes/70/wr/mm7032e2.htm. Accessed 10 Mar. 2022.
23 "COVID-19 Incidence and Death Rates Among Unvaccinated". 28 Jan. 2022, https://www.cdc.gov/mmwr/volumes/71/wr/mm7104e2.htm. Accessed 10 Mar. 2022.
24 "Effectiveness of a Third Dose of mRNA Vaccines Against COVID-19". 28 Jan. 2022, https://www.cdc.gov/mmwr/volumes/71/wr/mm7104e3.htm. Accessed 10 Mar. 2022.
25 "Vaccine Efficacy, Effectiveness and Protection – WHO | World Health …". 14 Jul. 2021, https://www.who.int/news-room/feature-stories/detail/vaccine-efficacy-effectiveness-and-protection. Accessed 10 Mar. 2022.

19 Natural Disaster (Hurricane) as Health-Related Event in SARS-CoV2 Delta Variant Exponential Transmissibility and Mortality

Background and Significance

Natural disasters have been epidemiologically observed to lead to increased disease distribution and determinants at a specific population level. Currently, epidemiology reflects the distribution and determinants of natural disasters including, although not limited to, hurricanes, tsunamis, tornedoes, earthquakes, and the application of such data in the control and prevention of casualties, accidents, injuries, survival and mortality at the specific population and location levels. Specifically, as populations experience ecosystem and nutritional imbalance during hurricanes and earthquakes, human health especially among the undeserved and racial/ethnic minorities present with a disproportionate burden of injuries, disease and suffering due to limited access to care, poor care quality and outcomes.[1] Natural disasters predispose to adverse morbidity, prognosis and excess mortality due to ecosystem alteration and lack of nutritional resources in immune system potentiation, resulting in increased viral replication and infectivity due to immunoglobulins and integrative immune response (T-cells, NK-cells) downregulation.[2,3] Additionally, lack of resources such as health inequity, implying the unfair and unjust allocation of social, economic and environmental resources pertaining to health after a natural disaster predispose some subpopulations, namely Blacks/AA, American Indians and Hispanics in Mississippi and Louisiana, to the disproportionate burden of the expected damage from hurricane Ida.[4]

The current exponential spread of the SARS-CoV2 delta variant, while it is partly explained by misinformation and disinformation as well as cultural beliefs leading to vaccine hesitancy, restricted uptake and disproportionate mortality among the unvaccinated, natural disaster such as hurricanes and earthquakes remain a feasible explanation of the global COVID-19 delta variant pandemic.[5,6,7] With the variability in the delta variant, relative to the initial alpha and beta variants, this strain (delta) remains more mutagenic, implying the opportunity for exponential viral replication and infectivity as observed by viral load, which is 1,000 times as likely compared to alpha and beta variants. Specifically, vaccine hesitancy from vaccine-eligible Americans, and the unwillingness to receive this safe and effective SARS-CoV2 (COVID-19) vaccine, results in increased case positivity, ICU admissions and hospitalization as well as mortality.[8]

Without a reliable immuno-epidemiologic approach to address victims of natural disaster, as a risk and predisposing factor in pathogenic microbe infectivity, there will be an excess SARS-CoV2 seropositivity and mortality prediction, an addendum to SARS-CoV2 delta strain exponential spread.[9] Therefore, since natural disaster remains a pathway to exponential spread of any pathogenic microbe, an immuno-epidemiological response is to encourage all vaccine-eligible Americans to be vaccinated for community herd immunity attainment (75–85% of vaccine uptake).[10] Additionally, there is an instant need for a global approach, implying the WHO initiative for vaccine delivery in parts of the world experiencing a natural disaster, such as Haiti, as well

DOI: 10.4324/9781003424451-19

as the CDC approach to State of Louisiana and Mississippi, with hurricane Ida as category four, for COVID-19 tracing, tracking, testing and vaccine uptake for all vaccine-eligible residents in these states as well as the neighboring states (Texas, Tennessee, Alabama).[11,12]

Materials and Methods:

A qualitative systematic review as Qualitative Evidence Synthesis (QS) was used to examine published literature on the role of natural disaster in disease predisposition.[2] This QES recommends rapid vaccination of all vaccine-eligible Americans in Louisiana and Mississippi and neighboring states for community herd immunity enhancement, as well as the allocation of resources such as food and shelter for population density marginalization and immunoglobulin upregulation for T-cell activation and NK-cell integration.[6]

This QES aimed to: (a) explain the implication of natural disaster in viral pathogen predisposition, (b) observe the contributory role of vaccine hesitancy in the nexus between natural disaster and viral pathogen exponential spread with respect to the delta variant, and (c) provide immuno-epidemiologic perspective in the exponential spread mitigation and mortality marginalization.

This process involved the identification of peer reviewed studies based on sample size, objective, research question, design, analysis and inference. The search strategy involved: "viral microbes and natural disaster", "SARS-CoV2 and hurricane", "viral pathogens and vaccine hesitancy", "SARS-CoV2 Delta variant and spread/transmission". The inclusion criteria reflected only studies with full body text and not abstract as well as studies in English and Italian languages only. Studies with sample size <10 on non-experimental epidemiologic design were not considered in the evidence synthesis in this QES.

Results

The findings in this study based on the summary review as QES are observed below:

Implication of Natural Disaster in Pathogenic Microbe Exponential Spread

Epidemiologic data on disease distribution and determinants have implicated natural disaster in the web of causality with respect to predisposition and disease precipitation. This observation is clearly explained by increasing population density due to evacuation and population proximity.[12,13] The anticipated hurricane Ida landing of category four reflects the worst human potential impact of hurricanes in Louisiana since 1850. With this observation, residents of New Orleans, Baton Rouge and nearby cities and counties are required to evacuate to nearby cities, counties or states, resulting in increasing population densities in those geographic locations.[14] Since the delta variant is associated with 1,000 times viral load, immuno-epidemiologic perspective in viral replication and transmissibility urgently recommends evacuees of hurricane Ida to wear face masks and apply rigorous hand hygiene, as this population migrates to nearby geographic areas.[15] This face mask wearing remains a necessary requirement, since the anticipated damage, as observed by meteorological forecasting, may require weeks and months for the damage to return to the pre-Ida infrastructure and utility status.

The lower proportion of the vaccinated individuals in Louisiana (<40%) and Mississippi (38%) signals increased SARS-CoV2 positivity, increased ICU admission, hospitalization and mortality, with immuno-epidemiologic perspectives reflecting the need to vaccinate all vaccine-eligible residents of these communities in controlling the spread, thus achieving herd immunity. In natural disasters such as hurricanes, epidemiologic data observed healthcare providers shortage, especially registered nurses and nursing aides as well as medical supplies and hospital beds, implying limited access and marginalized quality care.[16] Therefore, if the residents of Louisiana and Mississippi states wish to protect the health of Americans in other states, there is a need for COVID-19 vaccination now in order to prevent SARS-CoV2 spread during hurricane Ida.

Since the immune system's potentiation requires antibody generation and the subsequent integration of T-cells and NK-cells in appropriate immune responsiveness, upregulation and immunogenicity, there is an urgent need to address this during natural disasters. This approach involves glycoprotein elaboration, since natural disasters limit the availability of balanced and healthy nutrients such as fruits and vegetables as well as sleep deprivation.[17] Specifically, there is a need for an organized effort for the availability of these nutrients to communities affected by hurricane Ida, namely these two states, especially Louisiana.[18] Therefore, in addressing delta variant spread, the US must apply disproportionate universalism in providing healthy nutrients and shelter, including sleeping supplies to the disadvantaged populations in the states of Louisiana and Mississippi. This initiative will not only mitigate delta variant spread in these affected states but all states across the nation, as well as address the health consequences of a natural disaster.[19]

Vaccine Hesitancy and Hurricane Driven Pathogenic Microbe Exponential Spread

Since no data are conclusive with respect to scientific inference or conclusion, all findings in science, medicine and public health are driven by some amount of uncertainty and hence inconclusive. Therefore, as scientific findings remain accumulative and dynamic, there is a need for all human populations to adhere to the current findings of Pfizer, Moderna and, to some extent, Johnson & Johnson vaccine safety and effectiveness in recommending SARS-CoV2 (COVID-19) for all vaccine-eligible Americans especially in Louisiana and Mississippi states for community herd immunity. With such initiatives, humanity moves towards the role of religion in science as reflected in the biblical notion of neighbors caring for neighbors. Therefore, if we comply with the biblical application of caring for each other, as we vaccinate ourselves, we are caring for our neighbors. While vaccine hesitancy is driven by misinformation and disinformation from social media and the historical context of syphilis in Black/AA communities in the US, immuno-epidemiologic perspectives reflect the application of current knowledge of these vaccines in vaccine uptake.[20,21] As the human population applies knowledge in health promotion practices rather than the historical experience of Blacks/AA in the syphilis experiment which was unethical, immoral and scientifically unacceptable today, vaccine uptake is necessary now. Therefore, for Blacks/AA in Louisiana and Mississippi, while we must maintain an appointment with history, this past should not determine our inclination for vaccine uptake but the current available data on the efficacy, effectiveness and safety of this vaccine in determining the health and survival of Blacks/AA in these states and the nation as a whole.[22]

Hurricane Ida Delta Variant Exponential Spread and Mitigation Recommendation

With the limited knowledge of immune system responsiveness during natural disasters, and the current SARS-CoV2 (COVID-19) vaccine hesitancy, this review, based on an immuno-epidemiologic perspective, recommends the following in not only addressing the exponential spread of the delta variant in this context of natural disaster, but the nation's exponential spread, ICU admission, hospitalization and mortality:

(a) Face mask wearing during the Ida hurricane and thereafter.
(b) Physical and social distancing for population density marginalization during evacuation, shelter and relocation.

(c) Vaccine hesitancy marginalization and increasing SARS-Cov2 vaccine uptake, compliance and adherence for all vaccine-eligible Americans in Mississippi and Louisiana as well as other neighboring states.
(d) State, county, cities and the nation's provision of resources such as supplies, accommodation/shelter, healthy and balanced food supplies and water for volume expansion, extracellular fluid for immune system potentiation and decreed viral replication, implying less severity, good prognosis and survival.

In summary, the scientific community, especially public health officials, require a collaborative effort with the healthcare delivery system, such as hospitals and clinics, in addressing delta variant spread during this hurricane, in ensuring that all residents in the states of Louisiana and Mississippi remain healthy. With this collective, collaborative and integrative initiative, we expect either spread stabilization or reduction rather than an exponential spread from the anticipated adverse effect of hurricane Ida.

Questions for Discussion

1. Explain the study design and the research questions and objectives in this study.
2. What is the epidemiologic design utilized in this systematic review? Distinguish quantitative systematic review from qualitative systematic review. Which of these designs allow for generalizability?
3. Explain the findings and the implication of these data in delta variant spread mitigation in a natural disaster.
4. Provide a public health recommendation in viral transmission marginalization during natural disasters.
5. Is natural disaster a health-related event? Explain its implication in specific populations and the potentials for disease control and prevention in this health phenomenon.

Notes

1 "Greater Impact: How Disasters Affect People of Low Socioeconomic …", https://www.samhsa.gov/sites/default/files/dtac/srb-low-ses_2.pdf. Accessed 10 Mar. 2022.
2 "Risk Factors and Risk Factor Cascades for Communicable Disease …". 6 Jul. 2018, https://www.ncbi.nlm.nih.gov/pmc/articles/PMC6038842/. Accessed 10 Mar. 2022.
3 "A Review of the Role of Nutrition in Immune Function – NCBI", https://www.ncbi.nlm.nih.gov/books/NBK230969/. Accessed 10 Mar. 2022.
4 "Environment and Health Risks: Of Social Inequalities – WHO/Europe", https://www.euro.who.int/__data/assets/pdf_file/0003/78069/E93670.pdf. Accessed 10 Mar. 2022.
5 "The Global Epidemic of the SARS-CoV-2 Delta Variant, Key Spike …". 30 Nov. 2021, https://www.frontiersin.org/articles/10.3389/fimmu.2021.751778/full. Accessed 10 Mar. 2022.
6 "COVID19 New Articles 25 Sept – Centers for Disease Control and …". 25 Sep. 2020, https://www.cdc.gov/library/docs/covid19/ONLY_New_Articles_25Sept2020_Excel.xlsx. Accessed 10 Mar. 2022.
7 "Covid Updates: Biden Receives Preliminary Report on Virus Origin". 24 Aug. 2021, https://www.nytimes.com/live/2021/08/24/world/covid-delta-variant-vaccine. Accessed 10 Mar. 2022.
8 "SARS-CoV-2 B.1.617.2 Delta Variant Emergence and Vaccine …". 28 Jun. 2021, https://www.biorxiv.org/content/10.1101/2021.05.08.443253v3.full. Accessed 10 Mar. 2022.
9 "The Global Epidemic of the SARS-CoV-2 Delta Variant, Key Spike …". 30 Nov. 2021, https://www.frontiersin.org/articles/10.3389/fimmu.2021.751778/full. Accessed 10 Mar. 2022.
10 "Herd Immunity – APIC", https://apic.org/monthly_alerts/herd-immunity/. Accessed 10 Mar. 2022.
11 "Rethinking Herd Immunity and the Covid-19 Response End Game". 13 Sep. 2021, https://publichealth.jhu.edu/2021/what-is-herd-immunity-and-how-can-we-achieve-it-with-covid-19. Accessed 10 Mar. 2022.

12 "COVID-19 Study on Scientific Articles in Health Communication – MDPI", https://www.mdpi.com/1660–4601/19/3/1705/htm. Accessed 10 Mar. 2022.

13 "SARS-CoV-2 B.1.617.2 Delta Variant Emergence and Vaccine …". 28 Jun. 2021, https://www.biorxiv.org/content/10.1101/2021.05.08.443253v3.full. Accessed 10 Mar. 2022.

14 "The Global Epidemic of the SARS-CoV-2 Delta Variant, Key Spike …". 30 Nov. 2021, https://www.frontiersin.org/articles/10.3389/fimmu.2021.751778/full. Accessed 10 Mar. 2022.

15 "Herd Immunity - APIC." https://apic.org/monthly_alerts/herd-immunity/. Accessed 10 Mar. 2022.

16 Rethinking Herd Immunity and the Covid-19 Response End Game". 13 Sep. 2021, https://publichealth.jhu.edu/2021/what-is-herd-immunity-and-how-can-we-achieve-it-with-covid-19. Accessed 10 Mar. 2022.

17 "COVID-19 Study on Scientific Articles in Health Communication – MDPI", https://www.mdpi.com/1660–4601/19/3/1705/htm. Accessed 10 Mar. 2022.

18 "Hurricane Ida And COVID-19 Are Dual Threats In Louisiana … – NPR". 30 Aug. 2021, https://www.npr.org/2021/08/30/1032441006/storm-ida-covid-19-surge-louisiana-mississippi-hospitals-vaccines. Accessed 10 Mar. 2022.

19 "Relief to Louisiana and Other States Affected by Hurricane Ida". 2 Sep. 2021, https://www.charitynavigator.org/index.cfm?bay=content.view&cpid=9005. Accessed 10 Mar. 2022.

20 "Governor Pritzker Announces COVID-19 Vaccine Requirement for …", https://www.illinois.gov/news/press-release.23808.html. Accessed 10 Mar. 2022.

21 "Why Statistical Inference from Clinical Trials is Likely to Generate False …". 22 Aug. 2017, https://bmcmedresmethodol.biomedcentral.com/articles/10.1186/s12874-017-0399-0. Accessed 10 Mar. 2022.

22 "Take the COVID-19 Vaccine. It's the Christian Thing to do – USA Today". 28 Jul. 2021, https://www.usatoday.com/story/opinion/voices/2021/07/28/take-covid-19-vaccine-its-christian-thing-do/5389873001/. Accessed 10 Mar. 2022.

20 SARS-CoV2 (COVID-19) Vaccine Effectiveness and Durability in Immunogenic-Related Comorbidities (Multiple Myeloma)

Background and Significance

The available literature in immuno-oncology clearly observed the immune system marginalized responsiveness following multiple myeloma (MM) diagnosis.[1,2,3] Specifically, as this malignant neoplasm is a tumor of the plasma cells, the building blocks of immunoglobulins,[4,5,6] the adverse immune response involves: (a) gamma immunopathies, (b) leukopenia and (c) thrombocytopenia. With the observed pathophysiologic mechanism process implication, there is increased risk of infections in MM due to leukopenia and compromised antibody generation following vaccination due to gamma immunopathies and leukopenia. While vaccines in general allow for antibody generation and immune system responsiveness toward immunopotentiation and marginalized pathogenic microbe transmissibility, pre-existing clinical conditions such as MM restrict vaccine effectiveness and durability. This observation is suggestive of all Americans regardless of pre-existing conditions to be vaccinated as long as such individuals are vaccine eligible and follow control and preventive measures in SARS-CoV2 transmission. Further, human society should consider scientific data in health decision making rather than depend on misinformation from social media and other sources in vaccine hesitancy.[7]

Pathogenic microbes such as SARS-CoV2, the causative pathogen for COVID-19, require control and preventive measures in mitigating exponential spread during the pandemic. Historical data on pathogenic spread clearly encourage community herd immunity in addressing pandemics and marginalizing the opportunity for mutations or novel variants, given viral replication and human host factors.[8] Specifically, this approach implicates immunization for all vaccine-eligible individuals in protecting individuals from infections, hospitalization, complications and mortality.

The current SARS-CoV2 vaccine has clearly observed effectiveness and decreased adverse effects among the immunized. These vaccines (Pfizer (mRNA), Moderna (mRNA), Johnson & Johnson (toxoid)) efficacy observed from phases I-III clinical trials allowed for the utilization of these data for the phase IV, implying community-based vaccine administration.[9] Currently, the effectiveness of these vaccines has been accurately observed despite the notion of scientific data remaining cumulative, indicative of the application of data dynamics in clinical and epidemiologic decision making in global vaccine recommendation in mitigating and eliminating the COVID-19 pandemic.[10]

While the purpose of any vaccine is to enhance antibody generation by the host immune system in hindering viral replication, not all individuals vaccinated are able to elaborate specific antibodies in neutralizing the SARS-CoV2 viral pathogen, resulting in immune complex generation as well as complement system activation initiated by C3, a critical complement system component in this neutralization process.[11] With the generated antibodies, T-cell activation,

DOI: 10.4324/9781003424451-20

namely CD4 as helper T-cells, become elaborated, thanks to antigen presenting cells (APCs) such as macrophages that elaborate monokine as interleukin I (IL-1) which binds to the CD4 cells for activation and further elaboration of the B-cells growth factor, namely IL-4, leading to sustained effective antibodies such as immunoglobulin. With these pathways emerged Natural Killer cell (NKC) activation and immune system integration.[12]

The bone marrow remains the origin of the B-cells as B lymphocytes that provided a humoral immune response – termed adaptive – while the T-cells are similar to B-cells in terms of the origin and specific immune response as adaptive.[13] MM is a malignant neoplasm of the B-cells. Specifically, the B-cells activation and differentiation results in plasma cells formation indicative of a high affinity of antibodies to a given antigen, implying host protection[14] from a presenting antigen such as a pathogenic microbe. While humoral immune response remains the function of the plasma cells, the rapid proliferation and somatic mutation of the B-cell receptor also leads to oncogenic mutations, as observed in plasma cell neoplasms including, though not limited to, MM.[15]

With the implication of MM in plasma cells as gamma-myopathies, downregulating antibody elaboration, implying increasing transmission, infectivity and complications, the current review aimed to examine the implication of MM in COVID-19 vaccine ineffectiveness, mainly increased transmission, complication and mortality from COVID-19.[16]

Materials and Methods

Design and Search Terms/Engine: A systematic review of literature was used to examine the possible role of MM in COVID-19 vaccine effectiveness and response to antibody elaboration following vaccine uptake or receipt. This approach utilized search terms and search engines mainly PubMed with English language as an eligibility criterion for a critical consideration of studies in this assessment. The search terms used were: "multiple myeloma and pathogenesis", "multiple myeloma and antibodies suppression", "vaccine effectiveness and hematologic cancer" and "COVID-19 Vaccine and multiple myeloma".

Eligibility Criteria/Data Quality: Studies with reasonable sample size, objectives, outcomes were assessed for inclusion in this qualitative systematic review. Also, studies published in English language only were considered for critical appraisal in this review. In this appraisal, the exclusion criteria involved the elimination of studies with abstracts only.

Data Quality: Only studies with reliable and accurate methodology were utilized implying internal validity prior to utilization in this review. Review studies were examined for the methodology applied prior to the consideration for assessment in the scientific statement or clinical opinion in this study.

Results: Synopsis and Scientific Statement

A critical assessment of the parthenogenesis of MM reflects the game-neuropathies, plasma cell dysfunctionality. Compared to T-cells, B-cells are derived from hematopoietic stem cells from the bone marrow. Hematopoietic stem cells differentiate into multipotent progenitors, common lymphoid progenitors, and eventually mature B-cells through the stages pre-pro-B, pro-B, pre-B, immature B, and transitional B-cells. The recombination activated genes, RAG1 and RAG2, physically recombine the variable (V), diversity (D) and joining (J) segments of the immunoglobulin genes. Specifically, RAG proteins work by recognizing and excising recombination signal sequences, which are conserved heptamer and nonamer sequences separated by a spacer. This mechanistic process leads to immunoglobulin heavy chain (IgH) D → J segments (pre–pro-B), and then V → DJ segments (pro-B). In effect if IgH gene is recombined, it then undergoes transcription, translation, and expression on the surface with a surrogate light chain, which triggers light chain recombination at the V $\rightarrow$ J segments, marking the pre-B stage.[17] This process first occurs at the kappa light chain and without a productive allele, then at the lambda light chain. Typically, surface expression of the paired heavy and light chains, termed B-cell receptor (BCR), is considered as the immature B-cell, and thereafter B-cell transitions the bone marrow into the periphery and secondary lymphoid tissues for B-cell maturation.

Due to the implication of MM in adaptive immune (plasma cells) response impairment, there occur frequent bacterial and viral infections within the respiratory and urinary tract system in patients diagnosed with this malignancy. While generalized and multiple symptoms have been observed in MM such as back pain, spinal discomfort, backache, nausea, vomiting, bone pain, shooting pain, fatigue, weight loss, headaches (high serum Ca level) and general discomfort[18] (anemia), etc., an estimated 33.3% of patients with MM present with no clinical features at diagnosis (routine laboratory blood work, gamma-immunopathy).

MM affects the differentiated B-cells and reflects a multifocal proliferation of clonal, long-lived plasma cells within the bone marrow (BM). The mechanistic process affects skeletal modeling, inducing destruction, serum monoclonal gammopathy, and immune suppression. Compared to most hematological malignancies, MM genomes vary substantially, implying MM genomes associated with several structural and numerical chromosomal aberrations and several mutations in a number of oncogenes and tumor-suppressor genes (TSG).[19]

MM as a malignant neoplasm is a tumor of the plasma cells, the building block of immunoglobulins, the adverse immune response involves: (a) gamma immunopathies, (b) leukopenia and (c) thrombocytopenia. The B-cells, or antibodies termed immunoglobulin, remain therapeutic as implicated by SIgA, IgG and other immunoglobulins. With this malignancy there remains immuno-suppression, impairing the adaptive immune system responsiveness to antigenicity. The observed involvement of MM in the white blood cells as leukocytes in infection, signals decreased protection from pathogenic microbes, including viral and bacterial. Additionally, MM impairs the platelet's functionality, resulting in thrombocytopenia as observed in bruises experienced by MM patients.[20]

The immune response in MM following vaccination remains marginalized due to the impairment in antibody generation, given antigenicity (vaccine). MM induces gamma-immunopathy which restricts adequate and durable immune response. Additionally, the observed immuno-suppression in MM results in decreased activation of T-cells as well as NKC integration in immune system responsiveness following vaccine uptake.

Discussion

This qualitative systematic review was motivated by the misinformation and disinformation on COVID-19 vaccine effectiveness in the US population. With the current misinformation of vaccine ineffectiveness among the elderly, especially those diagnosed with malignant neoplasm, we examined published literature on MM pathogenesis, especially the adaptive immune system suppression by this malignant neoplasm.[21] There are a few relevant findings based on these reviews:

First, clinical conditions such as malignancies, especially MM, suppress the immune system response. Second, not all individuals exposed to vaccines demonstrate vaccine effectiveness, especially the immuno-compromised and immuno-suppressed, implying booster shots and enhanced preventive and control approach for such individuals. Third, COVID-19 vaccine and other vaccines do not demonstrate comparable effectiveness compared to individuals without immuno-suppression, immuno-compromised and those with an organ transplant placed on immuno-suppressive agents.

Conclusions and Recommendations

In summary, immune-related comorbidities such as MM results in gamma-immunopathies, leukopenia and thrombocytopenia leading to suppressed immune responsiveness to antigen city including pathogenic microbes and vaccines. This review is suggestive of the application of control and preventive measures to all patients with MM vaccinated with COVID-19 vaccine, such as physical distancing, face mask and rigorous hand hygiene. Further, the COVID-19 complications and mortality among individuals already vaccinated is not explained by the ineffectiveness of the vaccine but by comorbidity such as MM. Based on this review, we recommend all individuals with malignant neoplasm to be vaccinated and adhere to preventive and control measures in viral transmissibility for community herd immunity enhancement.

Questions for Discussion

1. What is the research question in this qualitative evidence synthesis (QES)?
2. Describe the study design.
3. Explain the implication of MM in immune system downregulation and SARS-CoV2 transmission and COVID-19 complications.
4. Examine the findings and provide recommendations for future research in this direction.
5. What are the strengths and limitations of this study?

Notes

1 "Impact of Vaccines; Health, Economic and Social Perspectives – NCBI". 14 Jul. 2020, https://www.ncbi.nlm.nih.gov/pmc/articles/PMC7371956/. Accessed 10 Mar. 2022.
2 "What does Immunogenicity Mean in the Context of COVID-19 …". 19 Nov. 2020, https://www.astrazeneca.com/what-science-can-do/topics/disease-understanding/what-does-immunogenicity-mean-in-the-context-of-covid-19-vaccines.html. Accessed 10 Mar. 2022.
3 "Fifth-week Immunogenicity and Safety of Anti-SARS-CoV-2 …". 17 May. 2021, https://jhoonline.biomedcentral.com/articles/10.1186/s13045-021-01090-6. Accessed 10 Mar. 2022.
4 "Recommendations for Vaccination in Multiple Myeloma – Nature". 19 Aug. 2020, https://www.nature.com/articles/s41375-020-01016-0. Accessed 10 Mar. 2022.
5 "Efficacy of Covid-19 Vaccines in Immunocompromised … – The BMJ", https://www.bmj.com/content/376/bmj-2021–068632.full.pdf. Accessed 10 Mar. 2022.
6 "What Is Multiple Myeloma? – American Cancer Society". 28 Feb. 2018, https://www.cancer.org/cancer/multiple-myeloma/about/what-is-multiple-myeloma.html. Accessed 10 Mar. 2022.
7 "SARS-CoV-2 Vaccines in Patients with Multiple Myeloma – NCBI". 17 Feb. 2021, https://www.ncbi.nlm.nih.gov/pmc/articles/PMC7892292/. Accessed 10 Mar. 2022.
8 "Emerging Pandemic Diseases: How We Got to COVID-19 – NCBI". 15 Aug. 2020, https://www.ncbi.nlm.nih.gov/pmc/articles/PMC7428724/. Accessed 10 Mar. 2022.
9 "Coronavirus Disease (COVID-19): Herd Immunity, Lockdowns", https://www.who.int/news-room/questions-and-answers/item/herd-immunity-lockdowns-and-covid-19. Accessed 10 Mar. 2022.
10 "Statement for Healthcare Professionals: How COVID-19 Vaccines …". 11 Jun. 2021, https://www.who.int/news/item/11–06–2021-statement-for-healthcare-professionals-how-covid-19-vaccines-are-regulated-for-safety-and-effectiveness. Accessed 10 Mar. 2022.
11 "A Guide to Vaccinology: From Basic Principles to New Developments". 22 Dec. 2020, https://www.nature.com/articles/s41577-020-00479-7. Accessed 10 Mar. 2022.
12 "Helper T Cells and Lymphocyte Activation – NCBI", https://www.ncbi.nlm.nih.gov/books/NBK26827/. Accessed 10 Mar. 2022
13 "Lymphocytes and the Cellular Basis of Adaptive Immunity – NCBI", https://www.ncbi.nlm.nih.gov/books/NBK26921/. Accessed 10 Mar. 2022.
14 "What Is Multiple Myeloma? – American Cancer Society". 28 Feb. 2018, https://www.cancer.org/cancer/multiple-myeloma/about/what-is-multiple-myeloma.html. Accessed 10 Mar. 2022.

15   "The Rise and Fall of Long-lived Humoral Immunity: Terminal ... – NCBI", https://www.ncbi.nlm.nih.gov/pmc/articles/PMC2827865/. Accessed 10 Mar. 2022.

16   "COVID-19 Vaccination in Patients with Multiple Myeloma – NCBI", https://www.ncbi.nlm.nih.gov/pmc/PMC8553271/. Accessed 10 Mar. 2022.

17   "SARS-CoV-2 Vaccines in Patients with Multiple Myeloma – NCBI". 17 Feb. 2021, https://www.ncbi.nlm.nih.gov/pmc/articles/PMC7892292/. Accessed 10 Mar. 2022.

18   "Pathogen Recognition and Inflammatory Signaling in Innate Immune ...", https://www.ncbi.nlm.nih.gov/pmc/articles/PMC2668232/. Accessed 10 Mar. 2022.

19   "Pathogenesis of Monoclonal Gammopathy of Undetermined ... – NCBI", https://www.ncbi.nlm.nih.gov/pmc/articles/PMC3040450/. Accessed 10 Mar. 2022.

20   "The Plasma Cells | Canadian Cancer Society", https://cancer.ca/en/cancer-information/cancer-types/multiple-myeloma/what-is-multiple-myeloma/the-plasma-cells. Accessed 10 Mar. 2022.

21   "An Investigation of Misinformation Sharing by Subscribers to a Fact ...". 10 Aug. 2021, https://journals.plos.org/plosone/article?id=10.1371/journal.pone.0255702. Accessed 10 Mar. 2022.

21 SARS-CoV2 Omicron Variant
Transmissibility, Clinical Manifestations, Severity and Vaccine Effectiveness

Background and Significance

The SARS-CoV2 omicron variant is quite novel. The approach is to observe current data on what is the issue is with respect to this mutant transmission as well as its contagiousness.[1] Second, to address the gap comparing what is known and the application of such information in SARS-CoV2 transmission reduction and COVID-19 clinical manifestation management in order to improve prognosis.[1,2,3] With viral pathogens, which are not living organisms or cells, the more the mutations as observed in the current omicron variant, the higher the chance of immune escape resulting in infectivity, clinical complications and mortality.[1] Despite this observation, and the limited scientific data on this pathogenic microbe, the scientific community recommends the global community to be vaccinated and receive booster shots, return to control and preventive measures namely face mask wearing, social and physical distancing and rigorous hand hygiene.

Materials and Methods

A Qualitative Evidence Synthesis (QES) was used to assess published scientific literature on the implication of SARS-CoV2 omicron variant in increased transmission, infectivity and COVID-19 clinical manifestations and severity. This QES involved the identification of peer reviewed studies based on sample size, objective, research question, design, analysis and inference. The search strategy involved: "SARS-CoV2 delta and gamma variant"; SARS-CoV2 Delta and Omicron variant"; SARS-CoV2 Omicrons and COVID-19 severity"; "SARS-CoV2 Omicrons and COVID mRNA vaccine". The inclusion criteria reflected only studies with full body text and not abstract as well as studies in English and Italian languages only. Studies with sample size <10 on non-experimental epidemiologic design were not considered in the evidence synthesis in this QES.

Results

The findings in this study are indicative of the current SARS-CoV2 omicron and enhanced infectivity, COVID 19 complications, severity and mortality as well as the effectiveness of the current Moderna and Pfizer mRNA vaccine in transmission and COVID-19 severity. Below are the observed findings.

Omicron Variant Transmission and Contagiousness

The current data, although limited on genomic sequencing, on this pathogenic microbe is indicative of how contagious this variant might be. Relative to the first wave, beta, gamma and

DOI: 10.4324/9781003424451-21

delta, the omicron variant illustrates several mutations, indicative of enhanced contagiousness as well as immune escape. Specifically, as more data become available on this genomic sequencing, the transmission of this pathogen will allow the scientific community the opportunity to clearly identify how contagious this pathogen is.[4] The ability to very fully understand this contagiousness will depend on several data by subpopulation including, though not limited to, age, sex, comorbidity, vaccinated and unvaccinated individuals, etc.[5]

Omicron Variant Incubation Period and Infectivity

The incubation period reflects symptom manifestation following exposure to any pathogen, implying a progression from clinical, subclinical to clinical stage in a disease process. Data is not fully available in various locations or geographic locales of this omicron variant, requiring effort to accumulate this data in addressing transmission as well as contact tracing, tracking and testing.[6]

Omicron Variant Clinical Manifestations and Severity

Current data from the observed origin of this variant, South Africa, reflects less disease severity, which is yet to be confirmed but is unlikely due to the initial patients treated in South Africa who were young adults. As the patient population after infection becomes diversified in terms of age, reliable data on severity will allow for the observed clinical manifestation of this variant as severe, less severe or moderate.[7] However, based on the limited knowledge in viral pathogens mutations, it is highly likely that the omicron variant will present with severe manifestations relative to delta or other variants. We need more data in this area.

Omicron Variant Immune Escape and Vaccination

Immune protectiveness following vaccination depends on initial antibodies (immunoglobulins) that result in T-cell activation and NK-cell integration following vaccine uptake. With respect to the omicron variant, given more than 30 mutations, it is highly likely there will remain an immune escape, implying reduced antibody protection, resulting in omicron variant infection. With the observed immune system reduced responsiveness in this variant, it is highly likely that vaccinated individuals have the chance of being infected, however, the antibodies to previous variants will prevent disease severity and mortality.[8] Therefore, in order to observe the balance between the risk and benefits as a clinical decision making in pandemic mitigation and stabilization, the clinical-immuno-epidemiological perspective recommends all vaccine-eligible Americans, as well as the global community, to be vaccinated, which will increase community herd immunity and reduce the opportunity for another SARS-CoV2 variant.[9]

With the omicron variant, the immuno-epidemiologic perspective in community herd immunity recommends all vaccine-eligible Americans to be vaccinated with booster shots and the industrialized nations in the world to provide vaccines to the developing nations for global herd immunity.[10] Therefore, failure to address this global collaborative vaccine delivery to the developed nations, as well as the US and other nation's vaccine hesitancy, will render this pandemic a "continuum", implying global population size reduction, increased global mortality due to COVID-19 as the leading cause of death in 2021/2022. Additionally with the limited data on this variant, the WHO and CDC should recommend booster shots for all vaccinated individuals as well as return to the preventive and control measures in this pandemic mitigation, namely face mask wearing, social and physical distancing and rigorous hand hygiene.[11]

Omicron Case Fatality and Mortality

Historical data on viral case fatality and mortality signal viral contagiousness, clinical manifestations severity and outcomes complication including organ failure based in part on viral mutations. However, there is no data on these epidemiologic aspects which restricts observation of these aspects of the omicron variant.[12] We anticipate increasing genomic sequencing, especially in the US, in order to initiate data gathering in this direction, especially among the unvaccinated Americans following exposure and transmission of this variant.

Conclusions and Public Health Recommendation

In summary, the omicron variant remains a variant of concern, requiring more data in a careful approach towards its control and preventive measures. With or without available data, the scientific community in the immuno-epidemiologic perspective recommends enhanced global herd immunity through vaccines uptake, thus mitigating the opportunity for another SARS-CoV2 variant, a more contagious relative to omicron.[13] Further, there is a need to return to viral pathogens control and preventive measures by adherence to: (a) social and physical distancing, (b) face mask wearing and (c) rigorous hand hygiene for all vaccinated and unvaccinated individuals globally.

Questions for Discussion

1. Explain the design utilized in this study.
2. What are the research questions and aims?
3. What are the main findings? Do SARS-CoV2 omicron clinical manifestations in COVID-19 remain more severe relative to the SARS-CoV2 delta variant?
4. Examine the strengths and limitations of this study.

Notes

1 "The T Cell Immune Response Against SARS-CoV-2 – Nature". 1 Feb. 2022, https://www.nature.com/articles/s41590-021-01122-w. Accessed 10 Mar. 2022.
2 "COVID-19: Vaccines to Prevent SARS-CoV-2 Infection – UpToDate". 7 Jan. 2022, https://www.uptodate.com/contents/covid-19-vaccines-to-prevent-sars-cov-2-infection?search=vacuna+covid-. Accessed 10 Mar. 2022.
3 "Summary of Guidance for Public Health Strategies to Address High …". 11 Dec. 2020, https://www.cdc.gov/mmwr/volumes/69/wr/mm6949e2.htm. Accessed 10 Mar. 2022.
4 "SARS-CoV-2 Mutations and Their Impact on Diagnostics … – Frontiers". 22 Feb. 2022, https://www.frontiersin.org/articles/10.3389/fmed.2022.815389/full. Accessed 10 Mar. 2022.
5 "Medicare and Medicaid Programs; Omnibus COVID-19 Health Care …". 5 Nov. 2021, https://www.federalregister.gov/documents/2021/11/05/2021–23831/medicare-and-medicaid-programs-omnibus-covid-19-health-care-staff-vaccination. Accessed 10 Mar. 2022.
6 "Investigation of a SARS-CoV-2 B.1.1.529 (Omicron) Variant Cluster". 31 Dec. 2021, https://www.cdc.gov/mmwr/volumes/70/wr/mm705152e3.htm. Accessed 10 Mar. 2022.
7 "Science Brief: COVID-19 Vaccines and Vaccination – Centers for …", https://www.cdc.gov/coronavirus/2019-ncov/science/science-briefs/fully-vaccinated-people.html. Accessed 10 Mar. 2022.
8 "SARS-CoV-2 T Cell Responses Elicited by COVID-19 Vaccines or …". 2 Jan. 2022, https://www.ncbi.nlm.nih.gov/pmc/articles/PMC8781795/. Accessed 10 Mar. 2022.
9 "Interim Clinical Considerations for Use of COVID-19 Vaccines | CDC", https://www.cdc.gov/vaccines/covid-19/clinical-considerations/covid-19-vaccines-us.html. Accessed 10 Mar. 2022.
10 "Coronavirus Disease (COVID-19): Herd Immunity, Lockdowns", https://www.who.int/news-room/questions-and-answers/item/herd-immunity-lockdowns-and-covid-19. Accessed 10 Mar. 2022.

11 "Strategies for Addressing Vaccine Hesitancy", https://www.who.int/immunization/sage/meetings/2014/october/3_SAGE_WG_Strategies_addressing_vaccine_hesitancy_2014.pdf. Accessed 10 Mar. 2022.

12 "Insights to SARS-CoV-2 Life Cycle, Pathophysiology, and Rationalized ...". 12 Jan. 2021, https://jbiomedsci.biomedcentral.com/articles/10.1186/s12929-020-00703-5. Accessed 10 Mar. 2022.

13 "Omicron Largely Evades Immunity from Past Infection or Two Vaccine ...". 17 Dec. 2021, https://www.imperial.ac.uk/news/232698/omicron-largely-evades-immunity-from-past/. Accessed 10 Mar. 2022

22 SARS-CoV2 Omicron Variant Exponential Transmission and Mitigation Dynamics

Background and Significance

Viral pathogens remain genetic materials and not living organisms, requiring host factors prior to replication and survival. The pathway to viral survival requires careful adaptability in the host, agent and environment interaction. If the host in any viral infection is protected, exposure to such pathogens results in no transmission, implying no clinical manifestations, as observed in the natural course of a disease – pre-clinical, subclinical and clinical.[1,2] In effect, if herd immunity is not achieved (>80% vaccination) and the control and preventive measures are not effectively utilized, any viral pathogen remains opportunistic, resulting in several mutants and antigenic serotypes.[3] This viral pathogenic opportunity exposes the viral host of SARS-CoV2, human animals to exponential transmission with novel variants namely delta and omicron.

With the exponential transmission of the omicron variant, this qualitative systematic review (QSR) sought to: (a) assess the scientific data on exponential transmission and disease severity[4] and (b) examine the disease as clinical manifestation severity relative to the delta variant. Additionally, with the limited data on the current omicron disease severity, this QSR recommended pathways for omicron variant transmission mitigation.

Materials and Methods

A qualitative systematic review (QSR) as QES was used to examine non–peer-reviewed and scientific reports on omicron genomic sequencing, transmission dynamics and clinical features severity. The PubMed search engine was utilized while the search terms were: "SARS-CoV2 omicron and transmission"; "SARS-CoV2 omicron and COVID-19 severity"; "SARS-CoV2 omicron and clinical complications"; "SARS-CoV2 omicron and mortality". This approach involved the assessment of the study and scientific report objectives, study or sample size, outcome/s, analysis, subpopulation analysis and inference.

Results

While analyzing studies allows for evidence synthesis, all findings remain uncertain, implying sampling variability with random error quantification. The findings from this QRS observed the following:

(a) Omicron variant reflects an alteration or changes in the genetic code of SARS-CoV2 delta variant, with the main viral intent of enhancing its survival in the host cell over time. These genetic codes serve as the source for viral building including the spike protein for

DOI: 10.4324/9781003424451-22

SARS-CoV2. The current geographic locale on omicron variant data reflects two to three times infection frequency, compared to two days retrospective infection frequency. Specifically, if the infectious frequency of individuals in a specific setting within a geographic locale was ($n = 100$) on Monday, on Wednesday an estimated 300 were infected, which is indicative of exponential transmission of omicron variant. Omicron mutations had been observed to be more than 30, supporting this exponential transmission among vaccinated individuals.[5] Typically, there is a doubling rate of omicron variants every two to three days. However, increased mutation in any viral pathogen does not necessarily imply disease severity but is indicative of viral survival.

(b) With the observed several mutations in SARS-CoV2 delta variant resulting in omicron variant, the transmission rate is exponential due these mutations in the spike protein which provides SARS-CoV2 the opportunity to replicate in the host cell. The omicron variant is highly transmissible due to these spike protein mutations and remains opportunistic in escaping the natural antibodies among individuals infected with the delta variant. Additionally, vaccinated individuals experience transmission due to antibody limitation.

(c) Omicron clinical manifestations with the current data reflect less severity relative to the delta variant. With more data on hospitalization, ICU admissions and mortality becoming available, more observations on severity will emerge.

Conclusions and Recommendations

The global assessment of the SARS-CoV2 omicron variant is indicative of its exponential transmission relative to the delta variant, however, reliable data are pending on comparable severity, hospitalization and mortality. Since all conclusions in scientific evidence discovery remain inconclusive, dynamic and not static data application is required in clinical and public health decision making.

This QES recommends the following guidelines:

Testing, tracking and tracing during this holiday season prior to family reunion. This initiative allows for marginalized omicron transmission during the Christmas period and the New Year gathering. Regardless of fully vaccine uptake, indoor gathering requires reliable and appropriate face mask wearing, and if feasible physical distancing. All vaccine-eligible Americans and the entire human population must be fully vaccinated, implying initial vaccines and the recommended boosters for immune system potentiation, amplification and enhancement. As the omicron variant escapes the immune response with the current vaccine, booster uptake will enhance antibody durability, stimulating the helper T-cells activation and NKC integration for enhanced and balanced immune responsiveness in marginalizing the clinical manifestations and severity of the omicron variant.

Specifically, the current omicron variant requires the following measures as control and prevention:

- Reliable face mask wearing.
- Subpopulation and granular data availability on omicron variant – age, sex, pregnancy, ICU admissions, hospitalization, mortality, prognosis, survival.
- Ventilation and healthy indoor air quality.
- CO_2 indoor air monitoring with reliable devices for enhanced healthy air quality.
- Physical and social distancing.
- Allocation of safe and effective vaccines to the underdeveloped nations (Africa, Caribbean, India, Bangladesh, Nepal, etc.) by the industrialized and developed nations namely the USA, UK, France, Germany, China, etc.

• Healthcare system adaptability to the omicron variant, given inadequate cancer screening, surgical procedures, ICU admission and hospitalization for morbidities, etc.

Failure to address the current incapacitation of the healthcare system will imply an epidemiologic re-transition from chronic disease to infectious disease as in a century ago. With the observed healthcare system incapacitation nationally and globally, if we as a human society fail to adhere to these SARS-CoV2 corona viral disease control and preventive measures recommendations including, although not limited to, full vaccine uptake, sooner or later the entire world will re-transition to infectious disease as the leading cause of mortality and epidemiologic re-transition. Realistically, the scientific community, based on this limited knowledge of the SARS-CoV2 (COVID-19) pandemic, must act now by informing the world community as a global village on a reliable and pragmatic approach to returning the human population to the pre-pandemic era.

Questions for Discussion

1. Explain the design utilized in this study.
2. What are the research questions and aims?
3. What are the main findings?
4. Examine the strengths and limitations of this study.
5. In future pandemics what recommendations should be applied in vaccine development following novel variants, such as gamma, delta and omicron?

Notes

1 "Estimation of Exponential Growth Rate and Basic Reproduction ...". 16 Jul. 2020, https://idpjournal. biomedcentral.com/articles/10.1186/s40249-020-00718-y. Accessed 11 Mar. 2022.
2 "The Immune System – NCBI". 26 Oct. 2016, https://www.ncbi.nlm.nih.gov/pmc/articles/ PMC5091071/. Accessed 11 Mar. 2022.
3 "Rethinking Herd Immunity and the Covid-19 Response End Game". 13 Sep. 2021, https://publichealth. jhu.edu/2021/what-is-herd-immunity-and-how-can-we-achieve-it-with-covid-19. Accessed 11 Mar. 2022.
4 "Potential Rapid Increase of Omicron Variant Infections in the United ...". 20 Dec. 2021, https://www. cdc.gov/coronavirus/2019-ncov/science/forecasting/mathematical-modeling-outbreak.html. Accessed 11 Mar. 2022.
5 "Enhancing Response to Omicron SARS-CoV-2 Variant – WHO | World ...", https://www.who. int/publications/m/item/enhancing-readiness-for-omicron-(b.1.1.529)-technical-brief-and-priority-actions-for-member-states. Accessed 11 Mar. 2022.

23 SARS-CoV2 (COVID-19) Morbidity Implication in Chronic Disease (Type II Diabetes – T2D) and Pancreatic Carcinoma

Background and Significance

Viral pathogens such as CMV, influenza A, herpes simplex and hepatitis C infections have been implicated in decreased insulin sensitivity (IS) and increased insulin resistance (IR). Similarly, these pathogenic microbes increased T2D incidence and complications. SARS-CoV2 as a COVID-19 causative pathogen, has been observed in increased risk and incidence of T2D among children and adults. While data are not currently available on the precise mechanistic process, SARS-CoV2 viral infection in T2D incidence may be explained by excess pro-inflammatory cytokine elaboration (cytokine storm), resulting in increased IR and decreased IS, leading to glucose intolerance and T2D.

The current (second week in January, 2022) weekly moving average of COVID-19 incidence (709,633, implying 76% increase a week ago); hospitalization (141,385 (37%)) and mortality incidence (1,615 (29%)), and the vaccination prevalence of 62.5% is indicative of the need to examine COVID-19 complications and long-term effect upon treatment and recovery. Viral pathogenic microbe infectivity and clinical manifestations, historically and currently, have been observed with chronic diseases, following treatment and recovery. SARS-CoV2, a causative pathogen in pediatric COVID-19 as well as in the adult subpopulation, has been connected to an increase in type II diabetes (T2D), however, the precise mechanism of this clinical condition is not fully understood, requiring molecular assessment as well as clinical guidelines and therapeutics.[1, 2] Since this pathogen, especially the delta variant, had been observed with multiple organ compromisation due to marginalized perfusion in some patients, the implication of increased incidence in T2D among children infected with this viral pathogen may be due, in part, to decreased availability of the beta cells and insulin receptors in the pancreas, required for insulin binding and glucose transformation to glycogen for hepatic storage and subsequent utilization for metabolic activities.[3]

Specifically, SARS-CoV2, a causative pathogen in COVID-19 morbidity, is associated with an increased incidence of T2D, which is explained in part by immune and endocrine system integration dysregulation, resulting in cytokine storm, decreased IS and increased IR, implying glucose intolerance and T2D. Additionally, this pathogenic microbe may result in increasing incidence of pancreatic neoplasm, a malignant neoplasm with the worst prognosis and excess mortality due to its late stage at diagnosis and marginalized biomarkers of susceptibility and morbidity. This malignant neoplasm remains the only malignancy with the prevalence (existing cases) observed to be lower than the incidence (new cases).

Currently, non-experimental epidemiologic studies, although incorrectly classified as observational studies, since all studies, experimental or non-experimental are observational, have implicated diabetes, a persistent and ongoing glucose intolerance, as cellular glucotoxicity in

DOI: 10.4324/9781003424451-23

pancreatic neoplasm and with the increasing incidence of T2D among children due to this pathogenic microbe, pancreatic neoplasm incidence will increase with this malignancy as the[4] only malignant neoplasm with a lower prevalence relative to incidence in any setting, due to lack of appropriate and reliable biomarkers and late stage at diagnosis. This qualitative systematic review (QSR) as QES attempts to examine viral pathogens (inflammatory process and immunologic response) associated with chronic disease manifestations such as T2D and the implication of COVID-19 in increasing T2D among children, especially pre-diabetics, as well as possible mechanisms for this implication (immunologic and endocrinologic mechanistic interaction). Further, this QSR, although inconclusive with respect to inference since scientific evidence discovery remains dynamic and not static, attempts to provide a clinico-epidemiologic recommendation in T2D incidence reduction affiliated with the COVID-19 pandemic in pediatric and adult environments.[5]

Materials and Methods

A qualitative systematic review (QSR) was used to assess published scientific literature on the implication of viral pathogens in chronic disease with specific focus on insulin sensitivity (IS), insulin resistance (IR) and T2D. Additionally, SARS-CoV2 and T2D remained a focused, although marginalized, data in this pathway to T2D incidence. This process involved the identification of peer-reviewed studies based on sample size, objective, research question, design, analysis and inference.[6] PubMed was the main search engine in identifying studies, with several search terms such as "SARS-CoV2 and T2D", "COVID-19 and T2D", SARS-CoV2 and insulin resistant", etc. The search strategy involved: "viral microbes and chronic disease", "SARS-CoV2 and chronic disease", "viral pathogens and insulin resistant", "SARS-CoV2 and insulin resistant". The inclusion criteria reflected only studies with full body text and not abstract as well as studies in English and Italian languages only. Studies with sample size <10 on non-experimental epidemiologic design were not considered in the evidence synthesis in this QSR.

Results: QES Synopsis

The QSR design in evidence synthesis as QES requires the observation of findings considered to be accurate based on the research questions, design, analysis and inference. The current result reflects the summary, synopsis and synthesis of the observed studies utilized in this QES as a brief scientific report for objective dissemination. The findings in this QES are categorized as presented below.

Viral Pathogens, Chronic Diseases (T2D) and Malignant Neoplasia

Immuno-epidemiologic data have historically, and till date, implicated viral infections such as influenza A, herpes simplex, hepatitis C, CMV, etc. in diabetes mellitus as well as Epstein-Barr virus in infectious mononucleosis and chronic diseases. Viral implications in T2D can be explained, in part, by aberrant insulin sensitivity (IS) resulting in insulin resistance (IR). Epidemiologic data have implicated marginalized IS in hepatocellular carcinoma, implying increasing incidence of this malignant neoplasm among patients with T2D.

The inert and adaptive human immune system responsiveness in viral infection involves pro-inflammatory mediators and cytokines as cell signals such as interleukin (IL) beta (IL-1β),

IL-6, IL-8 and interferon gamma (IFNγ) as well as tumor necrotic factor (TNF). The elaboration of these mediators in viral infections impairs IS, resulting in IR and glucose intolerance. Specifically, IL-6 had been implicated in suppressor cytokine signaling activation, resulting in marginalized IS. Further, INFγ elaboration from the natural killer cells (NKC) following viral infection had been observed in insulin receptor expression downregulation as well as IL-1β as a pro-inflammatory cytokine from macrophages, as antigen processing cells (APC) in collaboration with MHC-I in helper T-cell (CD4) activation and cytokine elaboration. Consequently, these cellular signal elaborations in these viral infections facilitate cytokine storms, resulting in <IS, and >IR and T2D incidence.[7]

SARS-CoV2, T2D and Malignant Neoplasia (Hepatocellular and Pancreatic Neoplasia)

While there is no specific data on SARS-CoV2 mechanism in marginalized IS and increased IR, T2D has been observed among pediatric patients with COVID-19 as well as adult patients. The observed increased incidence of T2D is explained, in part, by IS, IR, beta cells and receptor downregulation as well as the elaborated pro-inflammatory cytokines.[8]

Whereas viral infection requires IFN gamma elaboration, SARS-CoV2 was associated with marginalized elaboration among patients with severe manifestations. The observed IFN gamma adverse elaboration resulted in exponential transmission, severe inflammatory response, pneumonia, cytokine dysregulation, as well as pulmonary edema, neurologic dysfunction and hypercoagulopathy. T2D patients infected with SARS-CoV2 with severe clinical features were characterized with excess mortality relative to non-T2D patients. The increase in the hyperglycemic index among diabetic patients with COVID-19 reflects glucose dysregulation mediated by impaired immune responsiveness, thus enhancing cytokine storm.[9]

The observed incidence of T2D in the pediatric COVID-19 population is explained, in part, by pro-inflammatory mediators and cytokines as cell signals such as IL-1β, IL-6 and IFNγ as well as TNF elaborations. With these inflammatory mediators in SARS-CoV2 infections and COVID-19 morbidity, there remains impaired IS, resulting in IR and glucose intolerance, with T2D as a chronic disease.

While chronic hepatitis C infection had been implicated in hepatocellular carcinoma, the high hyperglycemic index in COVID-19 may result in hyperinsulinemia and glucose intolerance. With this molecular alteration, the beta cells of the pancreas reflect insulin dysregulation and the subsequent impairment of DNA replication, RNA transcription and mRNA translation, resulting in impaired gene expression, abnormal protein synthesis and cellular dysfunctionality. Whereas the exact pathway to pancreatic neoplasm incidence or development from COVID-19 is not fully understood, this condition may result in increased incidence of pancreatic neoplasm in future.[10]

Summary, Conclusion and Recommendations

Historical data on viral implication in chronic disease, namely T2D, clearly observed immunologic and endocrinologic interaction dysregulation. SARS-CoV2 and COVID-19 remain a predisposition to T2D, while a high hyperglycemic index remains to adversely affect the beta cells in the pancreas as well as insulin receptors, leading to pancreatic neoplasm, a unique malignancy, with an incidence rate higher than the prevalence proportion, due to late stage at diagnosis driven by inadequate and inaccurate biomarkers at the present time.

The findings from this QES although inconclusive, since all scientific evidence discovery are driven by uncertainties (random error quantification), is indicative of the need for the scientific community and public health experts globally to:

- Advocate SARS-CoV2 testing, tracing and tracking for diagnosis and treatment in preventing T2D incidence.
- Encourage all vaccine-eligible Americans to be fully vaccinated implying first and booster shots of Pfizer and Moderna for community herd immunity enhancement.
- Encourage the utilization of the pending FDA approval of the antiviral agent in symptoms management and immune system enhancement.
- Recommend the healthcare system to provide blood glucose evaluation for all patients with COVID-19 and SARS-CoV2 seropositivity.
- Encourage physical and social distancing.
- Require vaccinated and unvaccinated (ineligible individuals) to wear a face mask in any gathering.
- Advocate indoor air quality and ventilation in all settings.
- Encourage all seropositive individuals in any setting to be tested negative prior to community interaction.

With T2D in this pandemic remaining global in terms of increasing incidence, industrialized nations should allocate adequate and appropriate vaccines to the underdeveloped nations of the world as well as provide resources for the training of healthcare providers in these countries in appropriately delivering these vaccines to the poor and the undeserved in these global communities. Adherence to these observations and recommendations will allow for lower incidence of COVID-19–related T2D and the long-term effect of pancreatic neoplasm. While these recommendations remain inconclusive, the WHO and CDC should apply scientific data which are dynamic and not static in addressing TD2 and potential pancreatic malignant neoplasm during the COVID-19 pandemic.

Questions for Discussion

1. Explain the design utilized in this study.
2. What are the research questions and aims?
3. What are the main findings?
4. Describe the implication of COVID-19 in insulin sensitivity and T2D. What is the contributory effect of T2D in pancreatic neoplasm? Explain why some subpopulations with T2D are more predisposed to pancreatic neoplasm.
5. Examine the strengths and limitations of this study.

Notes

1 "Epidemiology of Viral Infections – NCBI", https://www.ncbi.nlm.nih.gov/pmc/articles/PMC7150207/. Accessed 11 Mar. 2022.
2 "COVID Data Tracker Weekly Review | CDC", https://www.cdc.gov/coronavirus/2019-ncov/covid-data/covidview/index.html. Accessed 11 Mar. 2022.
3 "Infection of Cultured Human Fetal Pancreatic Islet Cells by Rubella Virus", https://pubmed.ncbi.nlm.nih.gov/2648801/. Accessed 11 Mar. 2022.
4 "Rubella Infection and Diabetes Mellitus – PubMed", https://pubmed.ncbi.nlm.nih.gov/74564/. Accessed 11 Mar. 2022.

5 "Long COVID or Post-acute Sequelae of COVID-19 (PASC) – Frontiers". 23 Jun. 2021, https://www.frontiersin.org/articles/10.3389/fmicb.2021.698169/full. Accessed 11 Mar. 2022.

6 "Researchers Observed Association Between Standing and Insulin ...". 10 Sep. 2021, https://www.sciencedaily.com/releases/2021/09/210910121620.htm. Accessed 11 Mar. 2022.

7 "Influenza Virus-Induced Robust Expression of SOCS3 Contributes to ...". 16 Aug. 2019, https://www.ncbi.nlm.nih.gov/pmc/articles/PMC6706793/. Accessed 11 Mar. 2022.

8 "Interactions Between Diabetes and COVID-19: A Narrative Review", 15 Oct. 2021, https://www.ncbi.nlm.nih.gov/pmc/articles/PMC8554367/. Accessed 11 Mar. 2022.

9 "Role of Interferon Gamma in SARS-CoV-2-Positive Patients with ...". 4 May. 2021, https://gutpathogens.biomedcentral.com/articles/10.1186/s13099-021-00427-3. Accessed 11 Mar. 2022.

10 "The Effects of Type 2 Diabetes Mellitus on Organ Metabolism and ...". 22 Jul. 2020, https://www.frontiersin.org/articles/10.3389/fimmu.2020.01582/full. Accessed 11 Mar. 2022.

24 Ukraine Invasion and Global SARS-CoV2 (COVID-19) Pandemic Resurgence

Epigenomic Public Health Perspective

Background and Significance

War, which reflects societal instability, fundamentally affects the health of populations, including, though not limited to, risk factors exponentiation, marginalized tracking, tracing and testing, hospitalization, intensive care unit (ICU) admission, clinical manifestation severity, complications and excess mortality.[1,2] Additionally, with the departure of individuals and any subpopulation from the war zone to neighboring countries, such as Poland, SARS-CoV2 transmission remains global. Historical data on war outbreaks signal nutritional insufficiency and imbalance,[3] adversely impacting glycoproteins elaboration, the building blocks of antibodies – immunoglobulins. These antibodies initiate an adaptive immunologic response in any given pathogenic microbe's host exposure. Further, during the war, there remains an increase in population density as families migrate from the affected zones around the metropolitan/urban to suburban and rural areas, increasing pathogenic spread. Furthermore, compromised air quality increases pathogenic spread, especially viral such as SARS-CoV2 as well as pulmonary and respiratory system compromisation.

The Russian invasion of Ukraine, regardless of political differences, cannot proceed during any pandemic.[4,5,6] This qualitative review aims to observe the risk factors in pathogenic microbe spread during pandemics and recommend the pathways to invasion withdrawal in mitigating global SARS-CoV2 omicron variant spread and increasing mortality.

Materials and Methods

A qualitative evidence synthesis (QES) was used to examine published literature on the implication of war in public health as well as in disease outbreak and pandemics. The QES applies literature search and the PubMed search engine in examining published literature on the Ukrainian–Russian war and health consequences with specific focus on SARS-CoV2 transmission leading to COVID-19. Upon the application of quality criteria to the available literature, the articles that met the criteria such as objectives, clarity and conclusions/recommendations were utilized in this QES.

This research methodologic approach utilizes an epigenomic surrogate perspective, implying gene and environment interaction in this SARS-CoV2 and COVID-19 global pandemic resurgence. This initiative allows the understanding of how poor air quality, toxic water and air pollution impacts the innate immune system response, the T-cell and NK-cell integration with antibodies as B-cells or immunoglobulin in viral replication marginalization. Specifically, this QES observed the war related environment and the implication in human biologic system adaptation to antibody generation and integration with other organ systems such as endocrine, CVDs and neurologic in SARS-CoV2 transmission, as well as COVID-19 manifestation, severity and mortality.

DOI: 10.4324/9781003424451-24

Results – Synopsis

The synopsis in QES in indicative of the summary as synopsis in the observed literature. With the reviewed articles incorporated in this QES, there are reliable observations with respect to the current Russian invasion of Ukraine, namely:

(a) Compromised habitation and dwelling due to building destruction.
(b) Displacement of foreign medical students and students from other academic fields from the campus and their residents.
(c) Non-acceptance of racial/ethnic minority students, namely Blacks, as immigrants to Poland.
(d) Lack of food and nutrients across Ukraine due to these attacks.
(e) Departure of Ukraine residents to neighboring countries.
(f) Lack of control and preventive SARS-CoV2 measures such as face mask wearing, social and physical distancing.
(g) Unavailability of healthcare resources for COVID-19 treatment and management.

Discussion

This Qualitative Evidence Synthesis (QualLES) was performed due to the implication of disease outbreak and pandemics in war, and the potential for exponential SARS-CoV2 omicron spread, a COVID-19 causative pathogen, as well as public health and healthcare resources in spread mitigation, clinical manifestation complications and excess mortality, given this invasion.[7,8,9] This preliminary epigenomic surrogate public health assessment clearly observed the potential for nutritional imbalance, population density, healthcare resources and preventive and control measures in SARS-CoV2.[3–6]

Nutritional balance and healthy nutrition as well as lifestyle is required in reliable immune system response following exposure to pathogenic microbes such as SARS-CoV2. Additionally, the functionality of nutrients in enhancing immune system responsiveness for antibody elaboration depends on optimal temperature, which is adversely impacted in this invasion. With the observed adverse immune responsiveness, this invasion is required to cease in marginalizing the global COVID-19 pandemic. Population density impacts adversely on viral transmission, which is observed in this invasion. Viral dynamics reflect the close proximity of infected individuals in enhanced societal transmissibility.[3]

The control and preventive measures, if available and appropriately utilized, result in pathogenic microbe mitigation. The Russian invasion of Ukraine currently impairs and restricts access and utilization of face mask and social/physical distancing. Further, rigorous hand hygiene remains severely marginalized in this circumstance. Healthcare resource non-availability in this invasion signals comorbidities, indicative of increased infection as well as marginalized treatment and care for SARS-CoV2 infected individuals in Ukraine.

Conclusion and Recommendations

The Russian invasion of Ukraine is indicative of global SARS-CoV2 omicron resurgence and the opportunity for a novel variant. With the observed potential for the exponential spread of this pathogenic microbe, the entire world including, though not limited to, China, India and Iran must come together and recommend the end of this invasion for the benefit of humanity. This QES recommends these specifics:

(a) The United Nations establishment of a global public health committee in addressing the global allocation of health resources pertaining to the COVID-19 pandemic.[7,10]

(b) The WHO and CDC allocation of vaccines and resources for healthcare providers in the vaccine uptake for all vaccine-eligible Ukrainians, foreign nationals, and neighboring countries.

(c) The world community allocation of clothing, face masks and sleeping materials.[10]

(d) Healthy food allocations to all Ukrainians as well as foreign nationals and students.[7,8]

(e) Enhanced air quality for all Ukrainians, especially among those with a comorbidity such as COPD.[9]

(f) The urgent and instant acceptance of foreign medical students, especially Black females and males from other countries such as the UK, who are studying medicine in Eastern European countries because of low academic/tuition costs, relative to other Western European countries.

Questions for Discussion

1. Explain the design utilized in this study.
2. What are the research questions and aims?
3. What are the main findings?
4. Explain surrogate aberrant epigenomic modulations in health outcomes of the marginalized population during war. What is the WHO and global health recommendation during war in the viral pandemic era?
5. Examine the strengths and limitations of this study

Notes

1 Olha Zaliska, Oleksandra Oleshchuk, Rebecca Forman, Elias Mossialos. "Health Impacts of the Russian Invasion in Ukraine: Need for Global Health Action. *Lancet*, 2022, (10334); 399;1450–1452; https://doi.org/10.1016/S0140–6736(22)00615-.

2 UN Office of the High Commissioner for Human Rights. "Ukraine: Civilian Casualty Update 29 March 2022. https://www.ohchr.org/en/news/2022/03/ukraine-civilian-casualty-update-29-march-2022. Accessed 30 Mar. 2022.

3 WHO. "Health Cluster Ukraine. Ukraine: Public Health Situation Analysis (PHSA)—Short-form". 3 Mar. 2022, https://www.humanitarianresponse.info/sites/www.humanitarianresponse.info/files/documents/files/ukraine-phsa-shortform-030322.pdf. Accessed 29 Mar. 2022.

4 Yamey G, Arya AN, Bhutta ZA, et al. "A Call for an Immediate Ceasefire and Peaceful End to the Russian Aggression Against Ukraine". *Lancet*. 2022; (published online 24 Mar.), https://doi.org/10.1016/S0140–6736(22)00571-2.

5 Roborgh S, Coutts AP, Chellew P, Novykov V, Sullivan R. "Conflict in Ukraine Undermines an Already Challenged Health System". *Lancet*. 2022; (published online 11 Mar.), https://doi.org/10.1016/S0140–6736(22)00485-8.

6 McKee M, Murphy A. "Russia Invades Ukraine Again: How Can the Health Community Respond? *BMJ*. 2022; 376: 0548.

7 Southall DP, MacDonald R, Kostiuk O, Shcherbakov V, Deierl A. "The UN Must Provide Secure Medical and Humanitarian Assistance in Ukraine". *Lancet*. 2022; (published online 17 Mar.), https://doi.org/10.1016/S0140–6736(22)00526-8.

8 Sheather J. "As Russian Troops Cross into Ukraine, We Need to Remind Ourselves of the Impact of War on Health. *BMJ*. 2022; 376: 0499.

9 Murray CJ, King G, Lopez AD, Tomijima N, Krug EG. "Armed Conflict as a Public Health Problem". *BMJ*. 2002; 324: 346–349.

10 UNAIDS. "Global AIDS Monitoring 2019: Ukraine", https://www.unaids.org/sites/default/files/country/documents/UKR_2020_countryreport.pdf. Accessed 27 Mar. 2022.

25 SARS-CoV2 (COVID-19) Global Pandemic

"Extreme Epidemiology" Response in Transmission and Case Fatality Stabilization, Mitigation and Control

Introduction

Extreme epidemiology, a novel concept is the application of epidemiologic concepts and principles beyond the walls, "wall-less epidemiology" or epidemiology without borders, is comparable to "extreme causality" or "extreme medicine". SARS-CoV2, the causative pathogen in COVID-19 morbidity, remains a global pandemic, suggestive of a reliable scientific control and preventive measure response in flattening the epidemic curve and mitigating case fatality.[1] The utilization of what is scientifically understood about the risk of transmission, incubation period, clinical manifestations, management, and control, is needed now more than ever before in flattening the epidemic curve both nationally and globally.

Epidemiologic data reflects a transition from infectious disease as the leading cause of death in the 1900s to chronic disease, namely cardiovascular diseases (CVDs) in the current era.[2] This scientific experience provided substantial data to epidemiology on infectious disease modeling in terms of transmission, incubation period, subclinical disease, prognosis and fatality.[3] Additionally, epidemiologic approaches to infectious disease observed in the epidemic curve, could be due to excess fatality or transmission containment and mitigation through intense screening and pathogen detection.

The coronavirus termed COVID-19, a single-stranded RNA enveloped virus that enters the lungs via droplets and binds to Angiotensin-Converting Enzyme-II (ACE-2) on Type 2 pneumocytes for cell entry, is a particular antigenic type of coronavirus-disease causing pathogen, discovered in 2019, which remains a pandemic.[4] This microbe is an intracellular pathogen, meaning that it requires the host cells (humans in this case) in order to replicate and continue to survive.[1] The fatality proportion and not rate in the second week in March was estimated at 1.5%, lower than the estimate of 5.2% in late February and early March, due to the limited capacity in case detection which has moderately improved of late, with still more to be accomplished in the screening process. The global fatality proportion was 4.2%, which was due to the experience of 475 deaths in Italy despite the accelerated screening and preventive modalities in lowering the curve.[5,6]

This microbe, SARS-CoV2, is transmitted from person-to-person as a community-acquired pathogen. The mode of transmission includes viral droplets from the nose, eyes and mouth, with the droplet being able to survive on several surfaces over 24 hours. Individuals who are infected with this microbe may transmit the virus to others even though such individuals do not manifest any symptoms, these individuals are classified as asymptomatic.[7,8]

The clinical manifestations of COVID-19 include dry and productive cough, fever, sneezing, shortness of breath, tiredness as decreased vitality and lower respiratory tract colonization, including pneumonia.[9] Fever remains a protective mechanism for the host in order to limit

DOI: 10.4324/9781003424451-25

pathogen replication.[10] The early laboratory data on patients having fever and confusion admitted to intensive care units revealed hyperferritinemia, lymphopenia, elevated IL-6, C-reactive protein, and soluble CD25. These laboratory data are indicative of Cytokine Storm Syndrome (CSS). The CSS often results in acute respiratory distress syndrome (ARDS) and multi-organ failure resulting in increased fatality.[11] However, individuals could be infected with SARS-CoV2 without fever manifestation, especially if such individuals are immuno-incompetent, implying a compromised immune system response. The history of infectious disease is indicative of the limited clinical benefits of antipyretic agents in treating the fever of an infection. However, fever could be regulated in avoiding seizure, especially in children by low/moderate application of antipyretics, such as acetaminophen or paracetamol.[12] Specifically, the role of fever in infection is to protect the host by limiting viral replication via pathogenic transcriptome denaturation. The excessive use of antipyretics, for example in the context of a novel pathogen within the community without antibodies to the pathogen SARS-CoV2, is indicative of excessive viral replication and the inability of human interferon-gamma (INF-γ) to protect the uninfected human cells against the virally infected cells, and the subsequent cellular dysfunction and extreme community fatality.[13] This direction serves in part to explain the fever dysregulation in increased coronavirus fatality observed in Italy. Therefore, when the immune system is compromised, there remains an increased risk of infection and mortality, requiring immune system potentiation in epidemic curve flattening.

Materials and Methods

A cross-sectional ecologic design was used to assess the preexisting data on confirmed SARS-CoV2 (COVID-19) cases and mortality in March 2020 from CDC, WHO, Worldodomter, and STATISTA. A rapid assessment between March 23 and 31, 2020, was utilized for the extreme epidemiology response. The case fatality, termed fatality proportion, was examined using mortality in relation to confirmed cases involving the world, in particular, the US, UK, Italy, France, Spain, China, Germany, India and South Korea. The prevalence or proportion as cumulative incidence or frequency with respect to SARS-CoV2 seropositivity, case fatality and mortality was used to examine the population differentials during this period.

Results

The reliable sources consulted during the last week in March (23–31) reflected a global public health emergency and urgent need to flatten the epidemic curve in narrowing the unexpected outcomes of excess universal mortality and decreasing survival with COVID-19. With failure to adhere to pandemic epidemic curve flattening evidence-based practice data, as in the flu pandemic of 1918, such inadequacies result in the reduction of the world's population and the long-term effect associated with the economic crisis of COVID-19. The March 28, 2020 fatality prevalence or proportion, not rates were: Global (4.65%), USA (1.72%), UK (5.96%), Italy (10.56%), Spain (7.82%), China (4.03%), India (2.21%), Germany (0.5%), South Korea (1.50%) and France (6.05%) (Figure 25.1).

An increasing positive trend was observed on March 31, 2020 for the COVID-19 pandemic, with increasing FP globally and in all the countries: Global (4.81%), USA (2.00%), UK (6.40%), Italy (11.40%), Spain (8.80%), China (4.10%), India (2.80%), Germany (0.96%) and France (6.16%) and South Korea (1.66%) (Figure 25.2 and Figure 25.3).

The current (March 31, 2020) lowest fatality rate observed in Germany (0.96%) among the European countries and in South Korea (1.66%) is primarily due to "extreme epidemiology"

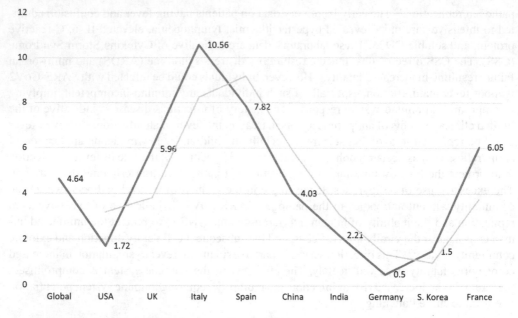

Figure 25.1 COVID-19 Pandemic Case Fatality, Globally and Selected Countries, March 28, 2020

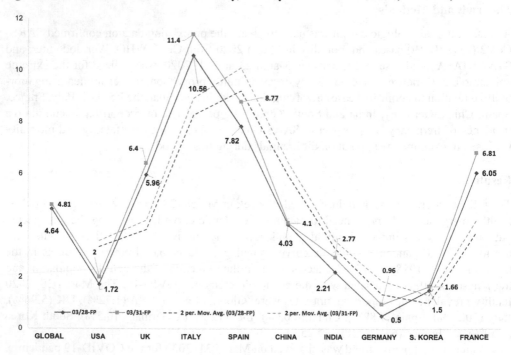

Figure 25.2 COVID-19 Global and Selected Countries Case Fatality, March 28 and March 31, 2020

response through the application of Wuhan, China, early data on COVID-19 transmission control measures and the effectiveness of the healthcare system in the application of resources (ventilators, trained healthcare providers, negative pressure rooms, decontaminants, personal protective equipment (PPE)) and adherence to the infectious disease protocol. The US fatality

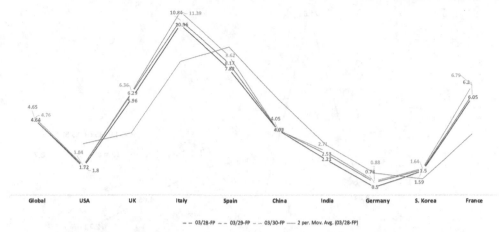

Figure 25.3 COVID-19 Case Fatality, Daily Trend, Global and Selected Countries, March 28–March 30, 2020

Notes and abbreviations: FP = frequency percentage; Mov. Avg. = moving average; 03 = March month.

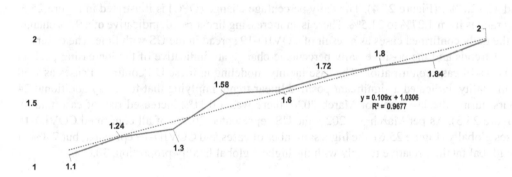

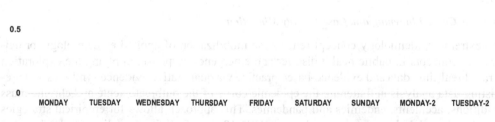

Figure 25.4 Daily Estimate of COVID-19 Case Fatality in the USA, March 23–March 31, 2020

Notes and abbreviation: R^2 = Coefficient of determination, implying the dependence of Y as outcome on X as independent variable.

proportion (FP) continues to increase due to improvement in screening and case detection, which is indicative of differential application of the strategies in Germany and South Korea, in mitigating the COVID-19 pandemic.

The US weekly FP observed this distribution estimates for the March 23 to March 31, M (1.10%), T (1.24%), W (1.30%), Th (1.58%), F (1.50%), S (1.63%), SU (1.80%), M2 (1.84%)

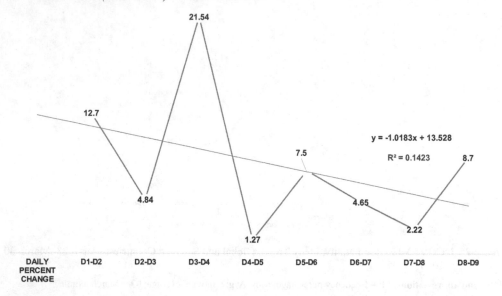

Figure 25.5 Daily Percent Change of Confirmed COVID-19 Cases in USA, March 23–March 31, 2020

and T2 (2.0%), (Figure 25.4). The daily percentage change (DPC) is illustrated in Figure 25.5, and ranges from 1.27% to 21.5%. There is an increasing linear trend, indicative of a 97% change in the daily confirmed cases as a result of COVID-19 spread in the US with time. The observed linear trends and the positive daily percentage change are indicative of the increasing peak in COVID-19 case confirmation. The case fatality modeling in these US confirmed cases as well as mortality, indicated a significant positive linear trend, implying that for every additional 24 hours during the last week of March 2020, there was a 0.11% increased risk of case fatality (Figure 25.5). As per March 31, 2020, the US represented 20.9% of all confirmed COVID-19 cases globally (Figure 25.6), the highest number of cases and COVID-19 epicenter, but 7.8% of the global fatality, relative to Italy with the highest global fatality proportion, 30.6%.

Discussion

Epidemic Curve Flattening and Case Fatality Mitigation

The extreme epidemiology concept reflects the mobilization of applied epidemiologic principles and concepts in public health disaster and emergency response, implying the exploration of rapid/real-time data and evidence-based practice via quantitative evidence syntheses and pre-existing data analysis in flattening the epidemic curve of the outbreak, acute and chronic mass conditions, accidents, endemics and pandemics. This approach allows for empirical strategies in addressing global pandemics, such as COVID-19, in infectivity modeling, epidemic curve flattening, and case fatality mitigation. The history of viral replication in infectious diseases indicates an epidemic curve with or without an intense response. However, flattening the curve in a timely manner reduces case fatality.

In ensuring a mitigated exposure and infection of healthcare providers in a healthcare system setting, the COVID-19 case detection, control and prevention taskforce guidelines must be utilized and should reflect: (1) facility decontaminants in reducing pathogens within the healthcare facility, (2) rapid isolation of symptomatic, suspected and confirmed cases and (3) healthcare professionals' protection from COVID-19 transmission. In mitigating microbe spread in terms of nosocomial viral infection, healthcare facilities should consider limiting the number of elective procedures or surgeries and reducing the number of entrances to the hospital facility, as well as ensuring that patients and visitors, such as patients caregivers or families, are screened for respiratory symptoms. The flow of patients to the hospital could be reduced by the hospital considering application of telehealth and telemedicine in providing care to patients. Second, healthcare facilities should initiate a properly ventilated triage environment, provide suspected or confirmed cases with a negative pressure room if feasible or closed private rooms with bath and aerosol-generating procedure (AGP) such as sputum induction, should be performed in an Airborne Infection Isolation Room (AIIR). Third, and highly relevant to such guidelines, is healthcare professionals' protection involving limited contact with patients at triage and confirmed COVID-19 patients' rooms and areas of care, rigorous hand hygiene, personal protective equipment (PPE) standard implementation as well as limiting the numbers of healthcare professionals delivering care to COVID-19 cases and prioritization of respirators and AIIR for AGP.

Conclusions and Recommendations

In summary, COVID-19 remains a pandemic, with the US as the current epicenter in terms of spread, while Italy remains the epicenter for case fatality. The observed transmission and case fatality pandemic require an Extreme Epidemiology Response (EER) to flatten the epidemic curve and case fatality reduction. Relative to emergency department (ED) response to an emergency and the emergence of extreme medicine from ED experience, extreme epidemiology (EE) is indicative of the need for a global initiative, especially the US healthcare system and public health department, to apply the available scientific data on COVID-19 transmission and case fatality, as well as adherence to the infectious disease control protocol (hand hygiene, PPE donning and doffing, negative pressure rooms, ventilators, and COVID-19 patient care room and treatment area requirements), intense case detection and contact tracing and testing as well as social and physical distancing. The inability to do so will not only prolong the epidemic curve

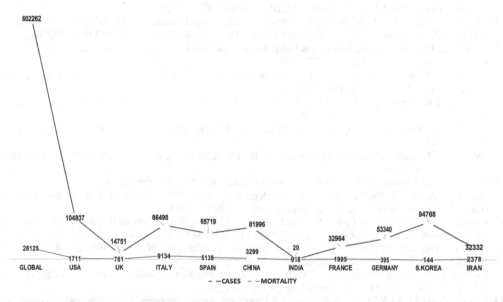

Figure 25.6 COVID-19 Confirmed Cases Versus Case Fatality Frequency, Global and Selected Countries, March 28, 2020

flattening but will expand the economic crisis related to COVID-19 spread, and hence exponential population expansion of socially disadvantaged individuals (low SES), increasing health disparities nationally and globally, adversely impacting world health. Specifically, COVID-19 transmission, if not addressed based on the available scientific data, will increase the US health data pool on health disparities, given the implication of social determinants of health in epidemics and pandemics.

Questions for Discussion

1. What is the research question and hypothesis utilized in this analytic epidemiologic study on SARS-CoV2 and COVID-19?
2. Describe the epidemiologic design utilized in this study and examine the data source.
3. Is this study a primary or secondary data assessment in SARS-CoV2 seropositivity and COVID-19 mortality?
4. What is the statistical analytic method utilized in these data assessments?
5. Are these data ecologic or individual level data? What are the limitations in the utilization of an ecologic data in SARS-CoV2 seropositivity and COVID-19 mortality parameter estimation?
6. What are the main findings in this study and the limitations of this study?
7. Is there confounding assessment in this study and the inclusion of such variables in a reliable parameter estimates with respect to the nexus between the independent and outcome variable? Was the effect measure modifier as a heterogeneity effect observed in this study?
8. Is the inference or conclusion reliable and accurate?
9. What are the suggestions or recommendation for future research?
10. Are the references appropriately cited?

Notes

1 Cascella M, Rajnik M, Cuomo A, Dulebohn S, Di Napoli R. "Features, Evaluation and Treatment Coronavirus (COVID-19)". PubMed – NCBI. Ncbinlmnihgov. 2020.
2 McKeown RE. "The Epidemiologic Transition: Changing Patterns of Mortality and Population Dynamics". *Am J Lifestyle Med.* 2009; 3(1 Suppl): 19S–26S. doi:10.1177/1559827609335350.
3 Jit M and Brisson M. "Modelling the Epidemiology of Infectious Diseases for Decision Analysis". *Pharmacoeconomics* 29.5 (2011): 371–386.
4 Aronson J, Ferner R. "Angiotensin Converting Enzyme (ACE) Inhibitors and Angiotensin Receptor Blockers in COVID-19". CEBM. 2020.
5 "Coronavirus Update (Live): 663,926 Cases and 30,880 Deaths from COVID-19 Virus Outbreak" – Worldometer. Worldometersinfo. 2020.
6 "WHO Director-General's Opening Remarks at the Media Briefing on COVID-19" – 11 March 2020. Whoint. 2020.
7 "Modes of Transmission of Virus Causing COVID-19: Implications for IPC Precaution Recommendations". Whoint. 2020.
8 "Coronavirus Disease 2019 (COVID-19) Situation Report – 51". Whoint. 2020.
9 Rothan HA and Byrareddy SN. "The Epidemiology and Pathogenesis of Coronavirus Disease (COVID-19) Outbreak". *Journal of Autoimmunity* (2020): 102433.
10 Evans S., Repasky E. and Fisher D. "Fever and the Thermal Regulation of Immunity: The Immune System Feels the Heat". *Nat Rev Immunol* (2015) 15: 335–349. https://doi.org/10.1038/nri3843
11 Mehta P, McAuley D, Brown M, Sanchez E, Tattersall R, Manson J. "COVID-19: Consider Cytokine Storm Syndromes and Immunosuppression". *Lancet.* 2020.
12 El-Radhi AS. "Fever Management: Evidence vs Current Practice". *World J Clin Pediatr.* (2012) 1(4): 29–33. Published 2012 Dec 8. doi:10.5409/wjcp.v1.i4.29.
13 Liu C, Zhou Q, Li Y et al. "Research and Development on Therapeutic Agents and Vaccines for COVID-19 and Related Human Coronavirus Diseases". Pubsacsorg. 2020.

26 Black/African Americans (AA) and Disproportionate Burden of SARS-COV2 (COVID-19) Mortality in the United States

Introduction

The understanding of the social gradient, implying the social determinants of health and health-related events, is essential in transforming health equity in epidemics and pandemics. Health distributions and determinants reflect social inequity, which is the unfair and unjust distribution of social, economic and environment conditions associated with health[1] resulting in health disparities and inequitable outcomes of morbidity and mortality.[2,3] Whereas smoking, reduced physical activity, unhealthy nutrients and excessive alcohol consumption have been linked to health outcomes due to decreased immune responsiveness and abnormal cellular differentiation and maturation,[3,4] the understanding of these determinants in infectious diseases, such as COVID-19, is relevant in epidemic curve flattening and case fatality mitigation. Epidemiologic data clearly implicate the subpopulations characterized by low education, low socioeconomic status, disadvantaged or deprived neighborhoods with excess morbidity and mortality in any epidemic and pandemic[5,6] relative to the socioeconomically advantaged.[7,8] Translational epidemiology that involves research at biologic, clinical correlates and population-based levels provides the perspective and challenges in addressing and transforming health equity during pandemics such as COVID-19.

Translational epidemiology requires a causal chain model in addressing epidemics and pandemics, which should be based on the social determinants of health (SDH), such as the conditions in environments in which people live, learn, work, worship, age and play. Specifically, these conditions reflect the availability of resources in addressing quality education, economic stability, health and healthcare needs, safe neighborhood and built environment, as well as social and community context.[9] These attributes of SDH reflect the social gradient in health, implying impaired health outcomes for the socially disadvantaged such as low socioeconomic status (SES) relative to the socially advantaged (wealth, income, high education). Available data on pandemic history, such as H7N9, implicate poverty, inequity and SDH in infectious disease transmission and the associated burden of morbidity and mortality.[10] The 2009 H1N1 influenza pandemic observed differential mortalities by socio-demographic[10] as well as substantial geographic variation[11] and population density.[12] In addition, the H1N1 pandemic observed an increased rate of hospitalization among the poor and those residing in poor neighborhoods as well as racial/ethnic minorities in the US.[13] Observed in the 1918–1920 flu pandemic, mortality was low SES as per-head income associated with healthcare access, care utilization, nutritional status and comorbidities.[14] A study on the flu pandemic in 1918 in Chicago observed significant disparities in transmission and mortality associated with socio-demographics namely population density, illiteracy, unemployment and age. Specifically, in relation to illiteracy, the multivariable

DOI: 10.4324/9781003424451-26

model after controlling for population density, homeownership, employment and age, showed a 32.2% increased mortality risk for every 10% increase in illiteracy.[15]

Blacks/African Americans (AA) as racial minorities are disproportionately affected by almost all pathologies in the US except tuberculosis (TB), cystic fibrosis, suicide, alcoholism and unintentional injuries as in motor vehicular accidents.[16] This population experienced excess adverse outcomes and morbidities, which had been attributed to social inequity and health inequity as exposure function of the SDH,[17] psychosocial stressors and unfair and unjust incarcerations. A recent review of race and 1918 influenza pandemic in the USA observed lower transmission (13% vs. 25%) among Blacks but higher case fatality (1–2% vs. 2–3%) relative to Whites.[18] The current COVID-19 global pandemic caused by SARS-CoV2, a ribonucleic acid (RNA) single-stranded enveloped pathogenic microbe, remains very virulent, with the potential to be transmitted by asymptomatic individuals or carriers. While population density increases the risk of COVID-19 as observed in New York City, Detroit and Los Angeles, race as a sociodemographic factor may play a role in transmission as well as mortality and higher case fatality among Blacks/AA compared to their White counterparts. Moreover, relevant to increased or differential exposure to SARS-CoV2 is low-income households, as reflected in Blacks/AA residing in apartment complexes and crowded neighborhoods in the US. The higher case fatality among Blacks/AA reflects the poorer health outcomes as observed in cardiovascular diseases (CVDs), hypertension, malignant neoplasm, diabetes, asthma, bronchopulmonary diseases, such as chronic obstructive pulmonary disease (COPD), and immunologic disorders.[19,20] These adverse health outcomes of Blacks/AA relative to their White counterparts reflect a lack of insurance, limited access to primary care providers and racial discrimination in the process of care navigation.[21,22]

Regarding viral spread, contact with the exposed individual, either symptomatic or asymptomatic as in SARS-CoV-2 increases the transmission, which explains the rationale for increased transmission and mortality among Blacks/AA who reside in dense population areas with crowded housing and suffer adverse environmental neighborhood factors, such as limited green spaces, recreational facilities, safe playgrounds and transportation systems. Blacks/AA relative to their White counterparts are more likely to use public transportation systems such as transit buses, which carry a higher probability of contact with infected COVID-19 cases, increasing the risk of infectivity among Blacks/AA.[23] Since a respiratory virus such as SARS-CoV2 compromises the airways resulting in acute respiratory distress syndrome, previous exposure to environmental pollutants and toxins precipitates poor prognosis. Such would be the case in a population associated with exposure to environmental toxins and pollutants, particular Blacks/AA.[24]

With evidence-based data assessment from pandemics and epidemics, reflecting higher case fatality among the socially disadvantaged, such as the poor, underserved and Blacks/AA (racial minority), this study intends to examine the current experience of COVID-19 in recommending urgent equitable preparedness in addressing mortality and case fatality in the US. With structural or organized racism as the main predisposition of Blacks/AA to excess pandemic mortality, the application of public health disproportionate universalism that mandates equitable allocation of resources necessary for optimal health and enhanced survival should be urgently implemented. The assessment of these variables such as income, SES, health insurance, safe neighborhood environment, access and utilization of quality healthcare, and lifestyles such as smoking, vaping, alcohol, drugs, physical inactivity, which are implicitly driven by structural racism, allow for effective intervention mapping in addressing what is "avoidable" and "unacceptable", social inequity as an exposure function of health inequities and disparities in morbidity and mortality.

The pathogenicity and virulence of a microbe depends on its ability to bridge the innate and adaptive immune response. The subpopulations with exposure to circumstances, such as food insecurity, psychosocial stressors and chronic morbidity have an increased propensity for viral transmission and infectivity complication, resulting in increased mortality and case fatality. Within the Black/AA communities, these exposures, in addition to the lack of health insurance, render the immune system incompetent through several mechanisms. An example of such a mechanism refers to the propagation of the conserved transcriptional response to adversity (CTRA) gene, resulting in an adverse consequence on interferon system elaboration during viral infection and decreased antibodies such as immunoglobulin G (IgG) synthesis. In addition, patients' response to therapeutic agents, such as monoclonal antibodies, anti-inflammatory and antiviral drugs, depend on transcriptomes, which serve as receptors to drugs or medications, or a lack thereof, which implies a decreased response to therapeutic agents.

This study aimed to assess the disproportionate burden of COVID-19 on Blacks/AA relative to Whites, explain the root causes, implying the social gradient and propose scientific and data-driven recommendations in narrowing the gap in case fatality between Whites and Blacks/AA. Specifically, we sought to: (a) examine the frequency of confirmed cases in the US and, by region and states, namely Illinois, Michigan, Louisiana, Wisconsin, Maryland, New York and California, (b) assess the cumulative incidence (CmI) of COVID-19 mortality by race and (c) determine the case fatality differentials between Blacks/AA and Whites.

Materials and Methods

This study was proposed to examine the exposure function of race as a socio-demographic factor associated with COVID-19 transmission, mortality and case fatality, with the intent to make recommendations for equitable resources during infectious disease epidemics and pandemics. With this initiative epidemic curve flattening and case fatality mitigation remains the norm in a pandemic in the US.

Study Design, Data Source and Variables Ascertainment

Data simulation and cross-sectional ecologic design was used to assess aggregate data on COVID-19 in selected states (WI, MI, LU, IL, MD, NC, NJ, NY, CA) by race. This design allows for an assessment on the correlation between the frequency of COVID-19 confirmed cases, mortality, case fatality and race. Data simulation was performed using data from the 2009 H1N1 outbreak with signal amplification and specific risk stratification by race. The data on risk modeling were available on the following states, namely WI, MI, LU, IL, MD.

The population of interest were geographic clusters by geographic locale such as states and race. These states were selected based on previous studies on the H1N1 influenza pandemic and the observed health disparities, with Blacks/AA representing the subpopulation with highest morbidity and mortality. The data sources utilized were the State Department of Health that provide COVID-19 cases and mortality by gender, county or location, age and race. However, these data, although reliable, were not very inclusive, since race data were not available for some COVID-19 confirmed cases and deaths.

Race as the exposure function of laboratory confirmed cases of SARS-CoV2 with ribonucleic acid (RNA) sequencing high-throughput process and mortality was self-reported from all tested individuals, positive or negative. The confirmed cases were based on either state or private laboratory tests on the viral RNA antigen. Other variables available for public access included age, gender, hospitalization, recovered cases and location of cases such as county, city, state, etc.

Statistical Analyses

Data simulation involved the use of an immediate risk ratio to assess the 2009 N1H1 influenza pandemic data. This was performed by cumulative incidence risk. The ecologic or aggregate data on COVID-19 from the states' public access data was used to determine racial variances or differences in confirmed cases and mortality. The case fatality was performed using the formula:

COVID-19 deaths/COVID-19 frequency or confirmed cases × 100.

(1) To determine the racial trends in the case fatality, we utilized the percent change by race:

Recent case fatality (RCF) – previous or baseline case fatality (BCF)/BCF × 100.

(2) The burden of the disease COVID-19 as a ratio of the shared contribution of subpopulations to the overall mortality was estimated using the formula:

proportion or percentage of deaths in subpopulation within the domain/the US Census 2020 estimated percentage of the subpopulation.

(3) For example, if the proportion or percentage of death in population A = 46% based on the total number of deaths in the overall population, and the population size of that population (A) = 14%, the COVID-19 burden for that population = 46/14 = 3.3, implying a disproportionate burden of death in population A.

   The binomial regression model (BRM) was used to determine the risk of dying from COVID-19 by specific populations in the race category. This model remains adequate in predicting the risk of dying from COVID-19 and by race stratification. The BRM is based on the probability of dying in the populations of interest, namely Whites and Blacks/AA, and with Whites as the selected population in the reference group for the relative risk assessment, as the risk ratio point estimate or magnitude of effect. In this model, we predicted the risk of dying, given the race of the confirmed COVID-19 case. The response or dependent variable 'y' (COVID-19 deaths), with each value in the independent variable (race/ethnicity) representing the number of success (k-deaths) observed in 'm' trials. Assuming the probability of success (death) = π, and the probability of failure (alive) = $1 - \pi$, a link function was used to relate the risk of dying to a linear combination of the regression variable, including the constant or intercept on the y axis:

ln (pr (success (death) = 1/pr (success (death) = 0) = $\beta 0$ (constant/intercept) + $\beta 1$(race).

(4) For example, the risk of dying from COVID-19 among Blacks/AA was compared to the risk of dying among Whites for the risk ratio estimation using 2 × 2 tabulation (A/AB)/(D/CD), A = confirmed cases and COVID-19 mortality among Blacks, B = confirmed cases with recovery/survival among Blacks, C = confirmed cases and COVID mortality among Whites, while D is confirmed cases with recovery/survival among Whites. A/AB is the risk in the exposed, Blacks/AA, divided by the risk in the unexposed, Whites, D/CD. In terms of the interpretation, if the two populations are comparable with respect to the mortality risk, the risk ratio (RR) = 1.00, and if the risk is higher among Blacks/AA, the RR is >1.0, but if the risk of COVID-19 is lower among Blacks/AA, the RR is <1.0.[25]

   The type I error tolerance was set at 0.05 (95% CI) and all tests were two tailed. The entire analysis was performed using STATA, Version 16.0 (StataCorp., College Station, TX, USA).

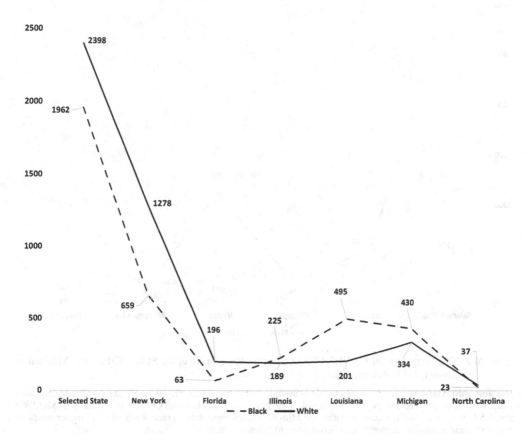

Figure 26.1 Frequency of COVID-19 Mortality by Race in Selected States, USA, 9 April 2020

Notes and abbreviations: The COVID-19 mortality frequency reflects higher occurrence in Illinois, Louisiana, Michigan and North Carolina.

Results

These data reflect confirmed cases of COVID-19 and mortality by race from selected states where these data are currently available. Although not in the table, the case fatality of SARS-CoV2, the causative pathogen in COVID-19 in the US as per April 14, 2020 was 4.11%, with New York, California, Louisiana as epicenters. As per 15 April, while the case fatality was 6.70% globally, the case fatality in the US was 4.94%.

The cumulative incidence (CmI) of COVID-19 mortality by race in selective US states and regions is illustrated in Figure 26.1 and Figure 26.2. The CmI of COVID-19 mortality in selected states and regions or cities with data on race reflects a relative increase in mortality of Blacks/AA with respect to population size, and Whites. These states were IL, LU, MI, NY, NC and WI (Milwaukee County). While Blacks/AA represent 13% of the population of the US as per US Census projection (2020), overall mortality was 34% (*n* = 19,062), with a 21% excess cumulative incidence of dying as per the April 9, 2020 data with a total death of 5,700. In the

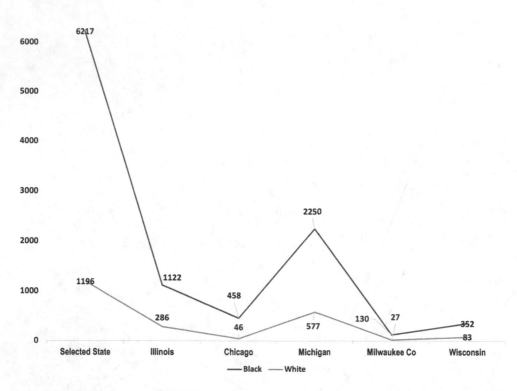

Figure 26.2 The Frequency of COVID-19 Mortality by Race in Selected States, Cities and Milwaukee County, USA, 9 April 2020

Notes and abbreviations: The cities with the disproportionate burden of COVID-19 for Blacks are Chicago and Milwaukee City as well as the county. These data reflect the cumulative incidence of COVID-19 mortality in Mid-West states, USA, 9 April 2020. Co = county; within the Mid-West states these data on race is indicative of higher mortality cumulative incidence (CmI) among Blacks/AA relative to Whites.

limited data on mortality by race, while Blacks represent 6% of the CA population size, the mortality data indicated 8% ($n = 21$). With the population size of Blacks/AA in LA County (8%), excess mortality was observed by the reported 16 deaths (17%). Similarly, whereas Blacks/AA represent 16% of the FL population, the mortality from the limited data, $n = 318$ (race/ethnicity data not available, 354–318) was 20% among Blacks, $n = 63$.

In the state of Illinois, Blacks/AA represent an estimated 14% of the total population but the CmI was 46%, $n = 225$. The population of Blacks/AA in Chicago is 29% but the mortality from COVID-19 was 70% ($n = 132$). Blacks/AA comprise 32% of the Louisiana state population but represented 71% ($n = 495$) of the total deaths ($n = 702$). The Black/AA in Michigan constitute 14% of the total population but the mortality was 53% ($n = 430$).

In NY state, Blacks/AA comprised 16% of the total population but illustrated 22% of mortality ($n = 659$). Similarly, while Latino constituted an estimated 19% of the NY state residents, there was a 24% ($n = 714$) mortality CmI. In contrast, whereas the population size of non-Hispanic or non-Latino Whites in NY state is 55%, the CmI was 43% ($n = 1,278$) of the total deaths, $n = 2,940$, which is different from the total deaths as per April 9, 2020, since race and ethnicity data were not available in most cases (7,067–2,940 cases). In NY city, Blacks/AA

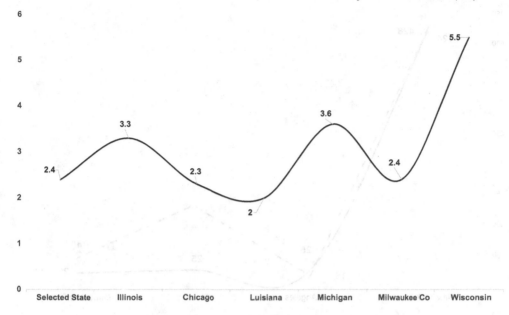

Figure 26.3 Disproportionate Magnitude of COVID-19 Mortality on Blacks/AA in Selected States and Counties, 9–13 April 2020

Notes: The point estimates on the line indicates the burden of COVID-19 mortality in the Black/AA communities in these geographic locales. As per mid-April 2020, the COVID-19 disproportionate burden of dying was outstanding in Wisconsin, Michigan and Illinois (Mid-Western states).

represent 24% of the total population, but mortality was 28% ($n = 428$), while Latino constitute an estimated 29% of the population but mortality was 34%.

In North Carolina, Blacks/AA represent 21% of the total population but the CmI of mortality was 38%, $n = 23$. The population size of Blacks/AA in Milwaukee County is 26%, but the CmI was 66% ($n = 45$). Michigan remains the third epicenter for COVID-19 next to New Jersey, with New York as the number one epicenter in the US. The case fatality in MI as per 15 April was 6.66%, while that of Detroit, the leading epicenter with the highest proportion of Blacks/AA was 6.85%. With case fatality in the US estimated at 4.93% during the same period, COVID-19 mortality disproportionately affects Detroit and Blacks/AA in the city. The mortality proportion in St. John the Baptiste Parish, LU as per mid-April was 7.9%. This population is characterized by environmental pollutants as a result of proximity to chemical plants and refineries.

The frequency of deaths adjusted for the population size in the Mid-Western states is shown in Figure 26.2. With the available data on race/ethnicity, Blacks/AA represent an estimated 34% of the total US COVID-19 deaths but make up 12.5–13% of the total US population, indicative of the excess burden of this pathogen on this community of color in Chicago, IL, Milwaukee City, MI and Milwaukee County in the state of Wisconsin.

Figure 26.3 examines the excess ratio of deaths based on the population size of Blacks/AA. For example, in IL, Blacks/AA represent 14% of the total state population but the COVID-19 mortality was 46% in this population, indicative of the disproportionate share of the burden of this pathogenic microbe in this community of color. The risk of dying from COVID-19 comparing Blacks/AA to Whites is illustrated in Figure 26.4. With Whites as the reference population in this binomial regression model, the COVID-19 mortality risk was higher in the overall states selected and in all the four states and Chicago.

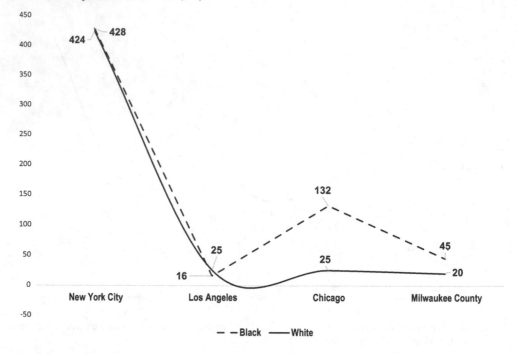

Figure 26.4 Black–White risk Differentials in COVID-19 Mortality in Selected States and Regions in the US, April 2020

Notes: The solid line indicates the risk of dying from COVID-19 comparing Black/AA with their White counterparts. With Whites as the reference group, implying 1.0 as no risk. In Chicago with a risk ratio (RR) of dying for Blacks/AA estimated at 2.24 in this model, implying that for every one death from COVID-19 among Whites in Chicago, more than two Blacks/AA experienced mortality from the COVID-19 pandemic.

Table 26.1 demonstrates the case fatality in the state of Maryland, stratified by race. The frequency of confirmed cases and mortality were 2,064 and 55, respectively, for Blacks on 4 April, with a case fatality of 2.7%, while the case fatality for Whites was 2.5%, $\chi^2(4) = 13.6$, $p = 0.001$. A follow up period by 4 April indicated increased case fatality among Blacks/AA, 3.3%, resulting in a positive trend in case fatality with respect to period change 22.2%.

Table 26.2 demonstrates the case fatality in Illinois, Chicago, Michigan and Detroit. In Illinois, the frequency of confirmed cases among Blacks on 9 April was 4,209, with 200 deaths resulting in case fatality of 4.8%, while a case fatality among Whites was 4.2%. In Chicago during 9 April, the case fatality among Blacks/AA was 4.5%, while among Whites it was 2.0%, $\chi^2(2) = 52.6$, $p < 0.001$. On 13 April there was an increase in case fatality in both races, with Blacks/AA bearing the greater burden of mortality. The case fatality in Blacks/AA was 5.9% and 3.2% for Whites, $\chi^2(2) = 110.8$, $p < 0.001$. The period percent change (PPC) for Blacks/AA was 31.0% and for Whites, 59.4%, indicative of a positive trend in mortality by these races. A racial variance was observed in CmI and case fatality in Michigan state. The case fatality for Blacks was 7.4%, while 8.0% was observed among Whites, $\chi^2(2) = 126.8$, $p < 0.001$. Although specific data are unavailable during this preliminary study, Detroit in Michigan illustrates case fatality disadvantage for Blacks/AA, with Blacks/AA relative to Whites observed to be 5.5 times as likely to die from COVID-19.

Table 26.1 COVID-19 Case Fatality in Maryland by Race, the 9th through to the 13th April 2020

Race	Confirmed cases	Frequency of deaths	Fatality proportion (%)	$\chi^2(df), p$
Maryland[1]				13.6(4), <0.001
Black/AA	2,064	55	2.66	
White	1,540	39	2.53	
Asian	122	6	4.92	
Other	449	3	0.67	
Unknown	1,354	21	1.55	
Maryland[2]				21.5(4), <0.001
Black/AA	3,202	104	3.25	
White	2,305	83	3.60	
Asian	190	8	4.21	
Other	861	12	1.39	
Unknown	1,667	28	1.68	

Data source, abbreviations and notes: Maryland Health Department, MD. AA = African Americans, χ^2 = chi square statistic, df = degree of freedom. 1 = Initial data on April 9, while 2 = data on April 13. The type I error tolerance, *p*-value was set at 5% (0.05).

Table 26.2 COVID-19 Case Fatality in Illinois, Chicago, Wisconsin by Race, the 9th through to the 13th April 2020

Race	Confirmed cases (n)	Frequency of deaths (n)	Fatality proportion (%)	$\chi^2(df), p$
Illinois				110.2(2), <0.001
Black/AA	4,207	200	4.75	
White	4,002	167	4.17	
Unknown	3,987	32	0.80	
Chicago[1]				52.6(2), <0.001
White	941	19	2.02	
Black/AA	2,102	95	4.52	
Unknown	1,450	7	0.48	
Chicago[2]				110.8(2), <0.001
White	1,209	39	3.22	
Black/AA	3,005	178	5.92	
Unknown	2540	15	0.59	
Wisconsin*				42.0(2), <0.001
White	1,726	83	4.81	
Black/AA	862	64	7.43	
Unknown	648	1	0.15	
Michigan				126.8(2), <0.001
Black/AA	8,460	625	7.39	
White	6,922	577	8.05	
Unknown	7,947	305	3.84	

Notes and abbreviations: 1 = Initial data on April 9, while 2 = data on April 13, 2020. χ^2 = chi square, df = degree of freedom, *p* = probability value for the random error quantification which was set at 5% (0.05) type 1 error tolerance. *Wisconsin reflects the assessment of the COVID-19 case fatality and mortality data from the Milwaukee City and County.

Although not illustrated in the table, Illinois state had a total number of confirmed cases, $n = 15,078$, mortality, $n = 462$, with a case fatality of 3.06% on Wednesday (April 8, 2020), while on Thursday (9 April) there was a case fatality of 3.22% (cases, $n = 16,422$, deaths, $n = 528$). As per US Census projection, 2020, Blacks/AA comprise 14.6% of the Illinois population, but represent 27.9% and 43.2% of COVID-19 confirmed cases and mortality, respectively. The Wisconsin data on 13 April indicate the total confirmed cases, $n = 3,428$, female $n = 1,817$ (53%) and male $n = 1,611$ (47%), mortality: male $n = 92$ (60%) and female $n = 62$ (40%). The Milwaukee County cases as per 13 April was $n = 1,743$, and 94 deaths. In Wisconsin, Blacks represent an estimated 6.7% of the population by the 2019 US Census estimate but constituted 25% ($n = 862$) of all the confirmed cases and 42% ($n = 64$) of all deaths.

Table 26.3 illustrates the Black–White risk differentials in case fatality with binomial regression models in MI, MD, IL, WI and the city of Chicago. The cumulative incidence risk of dying reflects the exposure function of race in COVID-19 mortality in these states and Chicago. There was a survival disadvantage for Blacks/AA with COVID-19 during the month of April 2020 in Michigan, with a significant 15% increased risk of dying relative to Whites, CmI risk ratio (RR) = 1.15, 95% CI, 1.01–1.32. In Maryland, there was a 5% increased risk of dying from COVID-19 among Black residents compared to Whites, RR = 1.05, 95% CI, 0.70–1.39. The state of Illinois observed a 13% increased risk of dying for Blacks/AA compared to Whites, RR, 1.13, 95% CI, 0.93–1.39. A 51% increased risk of dying was observed among Blacks relative to Whites in the state of Wisconsin, with most data from Milwaukee City and Milwaukee County, RR = 1.51, 95% CI, 1.10–2.10. In the city of Chicago, Blacks/AA were more than two times as likely to die from COVID-19 relative to Whites, implying that for every one White death from COVID-19, more than two Blacks/AA will die, RR = 2.24, 95% CI, 1.35–3.88.

Table 26.3 Black–White Risk Differentials in Mortality in Selected States, MD, MI, IL, the 9th through to the 13th of April 2020

State/Race	CmIRR	95% CI	p	EAF (%, 95% CI)	PAF (%)
Michigan					
White	1.00	referent	referent		
Black/AA	1.15	1.01–1.32	0.04		
Maryland					
White	1.00	referent	referent	5.0 (−42 to 36.5)	2.8
Black	1.05	0.70–1.58	0.81		
Illinois					
White	1.00	referent	referent		
Black/AA	1.13	0.93–1.39	0.22	11.7 (−1.0 to 28)	6.0
City/Race					
Chicago[1]					
White	1.00	referent	referent		
Black/AA	2.24	1.36–3.88	0.001	55.3 (25.5–71.0)	46.1
Chicago[2]					
White	1.00	referent	referent		
Black/AA	1.79	1.27–2.51	0.001	44.0 (21.4–60.0)	36.0
Wisconsin					
White	1.00	referent	referent		
Black	1.51	1.10–2.10	0.01	34.0 (9.0–52.0)	15.0

Abbreviations and notes: PAF = Population attributable fraction, EAF = Exposure attributable fraction, AA = African American, p = probability value for the random error quantification which was set at 5% (0.05) type 1 error tolerance. CmIRR = cumulative incidence risk ratio. 1 = Initial data on April 9, while 2 = data on April 13, 2020.

Discussion

With the current COVID-19 pandemic, and the US with the highest confirmed cases and mortality globally as well as the disproportionately observed mortality in some subpopulations, there remains an urgent need to examine these data, provide a possible explanation to the observed racial disparities and propose feasible recommendations in racial gap narrowing in COVID-19 mortality. Aggregate data were utilized from the various state health departments, where demographic information was available to determine the racial variances in the confirmed cases and mortality as well as risk differentials, comparing the Whites to the Black/AA subpopulation deaths. This preliminary study provides a few relevant findings to epidemic curve flattening and case fatality mitigation in the communities of color, namely Blacks/AA. First, of the limited data on race examined in the selected states and cities with race information, Blacks/AA despite the population size of 13% in the US, represented 34% of all deaths in the referenced states and cities. Second, there was a disproportionate burden of COVID-19 mortality among Blacks/AA. Third, the case fatality was higher among Blacks/AA relative to Whites. Fourth, Blacks/AA relative to Whites in all states and cities assessed for COVID-19 mortality had a higher risk of dying, implying excess mortality.

This study has demonstrated that, despite the 13% population of Blacks/AA in the US, this population represented an estimated 34% of all deaths from COVID-19 in mid-April 2020. The observed population variance and the highest mortality among Blacks/AA had been observed in recent media reporting.[23,25,26,27] The spread of pathogenic microbes, such as viruses, historically and to date has been linked to social inequity, where the socially disadvantaged populations convey the highest burden of the disease, including poor prognosis and mortality. The flu or influenza pandemic of 1918 through 1919 in the US observed a lower cumulative incidence of the disease among Blacks but higher mortality relative to Whites.[18] The current COVID-19 case confirmation among Blacks/AA mirrors the observed lower cases or morbidity among Blacks, due to decreased effort by the US public health system, local and county health departments and the healthcare institutions to provide the assistance needed such as transportation for Blacks/AA to access the screening centers and sites.

Second, Blacks/AA are less likely to be screened due to implicit bias[28] and lack of healthcare resources, including private insurance through well-paying jobs relative to Whites.[21–23] Clearly, the dynamics of viral pathogens reflects the penetrance in populations with compromised immune systems, driven by structural poverty and food insecurity, which Blacks/AA are more predisposed compared to Whites. With non-restricted conditions and the relaxation of clinical guidelines in infectious disease diagnosis during the pandemics, more cases are identified; isolated and contact tracing is performed for more screening. This effort lowers the transmission and the spread of the virus, enhances case detection, improves the prognosis and reduces case fatality at a population and individual level. Such initiative will reduce the unequal burden of morbidity and mortality now and in future pandemics.

Third, illiteracy rate and a lower level of education, which is higher in Blacks compared to Whites due to structured racism and racial residential segregation that deprived Blacks/AA of the opportunity of early childhood education, and quality early education had been observed to have an adverse effect on the transmission and mortality from influenza virus during the 1918 pandemic in Chicago.[15] Since Blacks/AA, historically had been perceived as a vulnerable population in pandemics and in COVID-19, the public health and the affluent societal identification of COVID-19 burden and engagement with this subpopulation of US society via national public health initiatives, will enhance a cooperative effort in data gathering and the understanding of the impact of a pandemic on the overall wellbeing of Black/AA populations across the nation.

The disproportionate burden of COVID-19 among Blacks/AA have been demonstrated in these findings. Besides this, SARS-COV-2 pathogen in COVID-19 and previous pandemics had observed similar burden as in the flu pandemic of 1918 and that of the 2009 H1N1 influenza pandemic.[14,15] The observed disparities and the disproportionate burden among Blacks/AA is explained in part by neighborhood-level social determinants, such as unemployment, educational level, housing and living conditions and population density.[7,10,29,30] The epidemiologic modeling of these factors provides reliable data in modulating these effects in anticipation of another pandemic, such as COVID-19. The social determinants of health as an exposure function of social and health inequities has been shown in the disproportionate burden in infant mortality, cancer, cardiovascular disease, stroke and diabetes among Blacks/AAs. These differentials, where Blacks/AAs are at a higher risk of diseases, reflect the unfair, unjust and inequitable distribution or allocation of social, economic and environmental conditions related to health. Additionally, the disproportionate burden of disease as observed among the socially disadvantaged populations, namely Blacks/AAs and Hispanics, reflects structural racism, which is different from interpersonal racism.

Racial residential segregation, the geographic clustering of racial and ethnic groups, has been observed to predispose subpopulations to health disparities[31] as observed in this study. Black neighborhoods in Milwaukee, New Orleans (LU), Houston (TX), Brooklyn (NY), Detroit (MI), and South Chicago (IL) are densely populated with apartment buildings. The spread of pathogenic microbes is enhanced by population density and close proximity as well as decreased hand hygiene and environmental conditions, such as contaminants. For example, St. John the Baptiste community in New Orleans, a Black/AA neighborhood, characterized by long-term exposure to environmental pollutants (chemical plants and refineries) represented one of the geographic locations with the highest case fatality in the US, 7.90% as per mid-April 2020. The long-term exposure to air pollutants has an adverse effect on bronchopulmonary function, resulting in chronic respiratory diseases, such as asthma and COPD. Specifically, the accumulation of air pollutants provokes the immune system response through innate and adaptive mechanisms. However, with persistent insult to the immune system adaptation, the host immune system remains incompetent with respect to macrophage activation and neutrophil migration, CD4 cells' activation and decreased cytokine elaboration, given macrophage inability to present the processed antigen or viral pathogen to CD4 cells for activation and B-cells or immunoglobulin growth factors' development and maturation. With COVID-19 implication in severe respiratory symptoms, populations exposed to long-term air pollutants are expected to present with poorer prognosis and excess mortality from this pathogenic microbe. However, the attributable fraction of exposed (AFE), given the environmental air pollutants in Blacks/AA neighborhoods observed in St. John the Baptiste community in LU, remains undetermined, pending the availability of sufficient data in risk estimation.

Additionally, the observed burden of COVID-19 morbidity and mortality in Black/AA communities is partially explained by workplace segregation, where Blacks/AA are employed in jobs with fewer or no benefits, but with more adverse conditions, such as buildings with no fire exit,[31,32] as well as a stressful environment. Specifically, Blacks/AAs who are employed as public transit drivers have an increased risk of contracting viral microbes, which also explains the COVID-19 racial burden differentials.

This study also observed higher case fatality among Blacks/AA relative to Whites. Previous studies in the flu pandemics of 1918 and 2009 clearly implicated the socially disadvantaged individuals and populations in survival disadvantage following infectivity.[18] The case fatality is a *proportion of those who died as a result of an exposure, divided by the entire exposed cohort as the population at risk for mortality, multiplied by 100* in a proportion and not a rate, and reflects viral symptom severity and poor prognosis from COVID-19. The excess case fatality among Blacks/AA is explained in part by the higher prevalence of chronic diseases, namely hypertension and other cardiovascular diseases, diabetes and cancer, as well as aberrant epigenomic modulation in COVID-19 prognosis and mortality. AA/Blacks are more likely, compared to their White counterparts, to be diagnosed with type II diabetes, primary or essential hypertension, stroke and cancer and have higher mortality from these conditions.[16] The higher incidence of these conditions among Blacks/AA had been associated with a lack of access to healthcare as well as decreased healthcare utilization due to several obstacles and barriers.[19] Second, the social determinants of health which reflect the needed resources to benefit from optimal health are not equitably available for Blacks/AA. These determinants are characterized by the social gradient upon which the socially disadvantaged individuals or populations are less likely to benefit from early education, quality education through college and a good paying job. The social determinants of health, namely education, socioeconomic status, income, employment, food security, racism, safe environment, insurance, transportation, and living conditions, adversely impacts the outcome of morbidity and mortality in Black/AA populations in the US.[33]

Since chronic health conditions render the biologic system vulnerable to microbes by compromising the immune system responsiveness, the observed higher case fatality among Blacks/AA is explained, in part, by the relatively higher prevalence of comorbidities among Blacks relative to Whites. While studies have indicated genetic polymorphism in the predisposition to hypertension as well as epigenetics and epigenomic modulations,[34] not much had been considered regarding the interaction of single-nucleotide polymorphism (SNP), epigenomics and the hypertension (HTN) genes involved in immune system regulation. Available genetic and epigenetic studies have implicated hypertension and cardiovascular disease candidate genes in immune system regulation, such as natriuretic peptide B(NAPB1), nuclear factor of activated T-cell (NFAT5), Human jagged 1 (JAG1), C-terminal Src Kinase (CKS), Lymphocyte-specific protein 1 (LSP1), adrenomedullin (ADM), auxin-binding protein 1 (ABP1), Feline sarcoma (FES), protein-tyrosine kinase (FES), angiotensin (AGT), serum/glucocorticoid-regulated kinase 1(SGK1), adrenoceptor beta 1 (ADRB1), nerve growth factor receptor (NGFR), cytochrome P450 family 1 subfamily A, member 1 and member 2 (CYP1A1, CYP1A2) and microtubule-associated protein 4 (MAPB4).[35] These genes mainly serve as negative regulators of B-cells (ABP1), suppress T-cell migration and activation (LSP1), reduce T-helper cells activities (ADM), downregulate innate and adaptive immunity (FES) and suppress T-cell proliferation.

The poorer prognosis and excess mortality of Blacks/AA with COVID-19 is, in part, explained by the highest prevalence of primary HTN and other cardiovascular diseases in this population, due to the candidate genes involved in immune system regulation that are implicated in HTN. In addition, it is not merely the gene candidates but their interaction with the environment that results in transcription factors or transcriptome dysregulation, which is necessary for immunomodulation. Addressing these health inequities will require the public health utilization of a disproportionate universalism approach where the population with healthcare needs are provided equitable resources in transforming health equity in the nation by environmental modification (toxic and air polluted neighborhoods, poverty, low income, illiteracy, lower education, violence, incarcerations, etc.).

Because Blacks are predisposed to more environmental pollutants and toxins, psychosocial stressors, a dangerous job environment and incarceration, these environments interact with the gene, implying impaired gene expression and increased disease development, poorer prognosis, increased mortality and survival disadvantage. In addition, because social gradient reflects environmental neighborhood characteristics, the understanding of gene and environment interaction, such as living conditions, may provide an additional strategic approach in intervention mapping for disease management and prevention. In effect, examining the gene and environment interaction, observed as epigenomics, will provide substantial data on intervention in narrowing the gaps between Blacks and Whites with respect to COVID-19 mortality.

Epigenomic modulations that commence at gametogenesis are transgenerational but reversible. The social signal transduction that is evoked from the stress placed on Blacks/AA has a substantial effect on the sympathetic nervous system and provokes the beta-adrenergic receptors. This response has been shown to involve the Conserved Transcriptional Response to Adversity (CTRA) gene expression and the consequent elaboration of pro-inflammatory cytokines due to the impaired gene expression of the transcription factors and the inhibition of gene expression with respect to anti-inflammatory response.[36] In understanding these pathways of genomic stability and their role in disease causation as well as mortality, epigenomic studies are necessary in determining whether or not Black individuals, relative to White individuals, have an increased mean deoxyribonucleic acid (DNA) methylation index with respect to the genome-wide analysis. Such initiative will involve the utilization of the bisulfite pyrosequencing that is very specific in differentiating between the methyl group and hydroxyethyl group, as well as the binding of these groups to the Cytosine-phosphate-Guanine (CpG) region of the gene, inhibiting transcription and the messenger ribonucleic acid (mRNA) sequencing, leading to impaired gene expression and abnormal cellular functionality. The reference to epigenomics investigation reflects the inability of a COVID-19 case to respond to treatment modalities due to the drug receptors in-availability, resulting from impaired gene expression (mRNA translation dysregulation).[37] The observed epigenomic aberration clearly illustrates treatment effect heterogeneity in which some subpopulations respond differentially to a given therapeutic agent in the phase of epigenomic lesion, explaining, in part, racial risk differentials in COVID-19 case fatality.

We have illustrated that in the states with data on race, Blacks/AA, relative to Whites, had an increased risk of mortality from COVID-19. The observed higher risk observed in mortality among Blacks/AA, diagnosed with COVID-19 and treated for the disease had been observed in other pandemics, namely the influenza of 1918 and 2009 N1H1.[18] With respect to the geographic locations such as states and cities, the risk ranged from 5% to more than twice as likely compared to Whites (CmIRR, 1.05–2.24). The observed excess risk of dying among Blacks/AA may be explained by the late detection of SARS-COV-2, implying poor prognosis, decreased access to identification and isolation resources, a lack of healthcare resources, and poor-quality care, where Black/AA patients are treated with implicit as well as clinician bias.[20,25,37] Also implicated in this excess risk are the social determinants of health as previously observed, where the socially disadvantaged individuals or populations are more predisposed to adverse health outcomes.

Despite the appropriate epidemiologic model used in this preliminary study to determine the Black–White mortality risk differentials in COVID-19, there are some limitations. First, this study used the only available data at this point, which is the aggregate data from the Departments of Public Health, which has a tendency for ecological fallacies. Second, there is a tendency for confoundability, since data were not available to assess and control for confounding in the risk estimation. Third, despite the sources of these data, complete race/ethnicity data were not available in these states and cities utilized in this risk estimation. However, the interpretation of these data remains accurate since an estimated >80% of the race/ethnicity data were available for this modeling. This preliminary study strongly recommends the collection and availability of race/ethnicity data from all states and US territories for the understanding of COVID-19 population dynamics for racial/ethnic minority populations' engagement and preparedness in the future, for health equity transformation in epidemics and pandemics.

Conclusion

Blacks/AA are observed with a disproportionate burden and increased risk of COVID-19 mortality compared to their White counterparts in the US, indicative of disproportionate universality in the allocation of resources for health equity transformation in future pandemics. Further, racial disparities in COVID-19 case fatality exist and will continue to persist unless data-driven scientific measures are implemented for racial/ethnic gap narrowing, thus reducing the probability and likelihood of COVID-19-2. The observed racial disparities are explained in part by social determinants of health (SDH), where Black individuals are exposed to environmental pollutants, social inequity, structural racism, food insecurity, poor housing and living conditions, illiteracy, low SES and a lack of healthcare resources. Likewise, aberrant epigenomic modulations remain a substantial explanation for the observed racial disparities in COVID-19 mortality in the US. These findings are suggestive of the need to apply public health essential services, disproportionate universalism, and social determinants of health in health equity transformation in future SARS-CoV2 variance. Efforts in that direction will ensure marginalization of opportunity for viral pathogens to replicate, induce manifestation, severity, as well as mortality. Furthermore, the application of these recommendations will guarantee global pandemic mitigation by the employment of disproportionate vaccine distribution and universal community herd immunity.

Questions for Discussion

1. What is the research question and hypothesis utilized in this analytic epidemiologic study on SARS-CoV2 and COVID-19?
2. Describe the epidemiologic design utilized in this study and examine the data source.
3. Is this study a primary or secondary data assessment in SARS-CoV2 seropositivity and COVID-19 mortality?
4. What is the statistical analytic method utilized in these data assessments?
5. Are these data ecologic or individual level data? What are the limitations in the utilization of an ecologic data in SARS-CoV2 seropositivity and COVID-19 mortality parameter estimation?
6. What are the main findings in this study and the limitations of this study?
7. Is there confounding assessment in this study and the inclusion of such variables in reliable parameter estimates with respect to the nexus between the independent and outcome variable? Was the effect measure modifier as heterogeneity effect observed in this study?
8. Is the inference or conclusion reliable and accurate?
9. What are the suggestions or recommendation for future research?
10. Are the references appropriately cited?

Notes

1 Samantha A. and Hinton E. "Beyond Health Care: The Role of Social Determinants in Promoting Health and Health Equity". *Health* (2019) 20: 219.
2 Owen WF, Carmona R, Pomeroy C. "Failing Another National Stress Test on Health Disparities". *JAMA* (2020) doi: 10.1001/jama.2020.6547.
3 Fiorati CR, Meirelles V, Elui C. "Social Determinants of Health, Inequality and Social Inclusion among People with Disabilities. *Rev Lat Am Enferm* (2015) 23: 329–336. doi: 10.1590/0104–1169.0187.2559.
4 Cooper G. *The Development and Causes of Cancer. The Cell: A Molecular Approach.* Sinauer Associates; Sunderland, MA, USA: 2020.
5 Crouse QS and Kumar S. "Health Inequalities and Infectious Disease Epidemics: A Challenge for Global Health Security. *Biosecur Bioterror Biodef Strateg Pract Sci* (2014) 12: 263–273.

6 Donkin A, Goldblatt P, Allen J, Nathanson V, Marmot M. "Global Action on the Social Determinants of Health. *BMJ Glob Health* (2018) 3 doi: 10.1136/bmjgh-2017–000603.

7 Cho HK, Lee SG, Nam CM, Lee EJ, Jang S-Y, Lee S-H, Park E-C. "Disparities in Socioeconomic Status and Neighborhood Characteristics Affect All-cause Mortality in Patients with Newly Diagnosed Hypertension in Korea: A Nationwide Cohort Study, 2002–2013. *Int J Equity Health* (2016) 15 doi: 10.1186/s12939-015-0288-2.

8 Walsh D, McCartney G, Collins C, Taulbut M, Batty GD. *History, Politics and Vulnerability: Explaining Excess Mortality in Scotland and Glasgow. A Report by the Glasgow Centre for Population Health, NHS Health Scotland, the University of the West of Scotland and University College London.* Glasgow Centre for Population Health; Glasgow, UK: 2016.

9 Center for Disease Control & Prevention (CDC). Social Determinants of Health (SDOH), Healthy People 2020. Available online: htpp//www.cdc.gov/socialdterminants/index.htm. Accessed 12 May 2020.

10 Szabo G and Saha B. "Alcohol's Effect on Host Defense". *Alcohol Res* (2015) 37: 159–170.

11 Wenger JD, Castrodale LJ, Bruden DL, Keck JW, Zulz T, Bruce MG, Fearey DA, McLaughlin J, Hurlburt D, Hummel KB, et al. "2009 Pandemic Influenza A H1N1 in Alaska: Temporal and Geographic Characteristics of Spread and Increased Risk of Hospitalization among Alaska Native and Asian/Pacific Islander People". *Clin Infect Dis* (2011) 52(Suppl. 1): S189–S197. doi: 10.1093/cid/ciq037.

12 Yousey-Hindes KM, Hadler JL. Neighborhood Socioeconomic Status and Influenza Hospitalizations among Children: New Haven County, Connecticut, 2003–2010". *Am J Public Health* (2011) 101: 1785–1789. doi: 10.2105/AJPH.2011.300224.

13 Deborah LD, Bensyl DM, Gindler J, Truman BI, Allen BG, D'Mello T, Pérez A, Kamimoto L, Biggerstaff M, Blanton L, et al. "Racial and Ethnic Disparities in Hospitalizations and Deaths Associated with 2009 Pandemic Influenza A (H1N1) Virus Infections in the United States. *Ann Epidemiol* (2011) 21: 623–630.

14 Murray CJL, Lopez AD, Chin B, Feehan D, Hill KH. "Estimation of Potential Global Pandemic Influenza Mortality on the Basis of Vital Registry Data from the 1918–20 Pandemic: A Quantitative Analysis". *Lancet* (2006) 368: 2211–2218. doi: 10.1016/S0140–6736(06)69895-4.

15 Grantz KH, Rane MS, Salje H, Glass GE, Schachterle SE, Cummings DAT. "Disparities in Influenza Mortality and Transmission Related to Sociodemographic Factors within Chicago in the Pandemic of 1918". *Proc Natl Acad Sci USA* (2016) 113: 13839–13844. doi: 10.1073/pnas.1612838113.

16 National Center for Health Statistics. "Health, United States, 2018" (2019). Hyattsville, MD. Available online: https://www.cdc.gov/nchs/data/hus18.pdf? Accessed 20 Apr. 2020.

17 National Academies of Sciences, Engineering, and Medicine. Health and Medicine Division. Board on Population Health and Public Health Practice. Committee on Community-Based Solutions to Promote Health Equity in the United States. In: *Communities in Action: Pathways to Health Equity*. Baciu A, Negussie Y, Geller A, Weinstein JN, editors. National Academies Press; Washington, DC, USA: 2017.

18 Økland H, Mamelund S-E. "Race and 1918 Influenza Pandemic in the United States: A Review of the Literature". *Int J Environ Res Publ Health*. (2019) 16: 2487. doi: 10.3390/ijerph16142487.

19 Garg S, Kim L, Whitaker M, O'Halloran A, Cummings C, Holstein R, Prill M, Chai SJ, Kirley PD, Alden NB, et al. "Hospitalization Rates and Characteristics of Patients Hospitalized with Laboratory-Confirmed Coronavirus Disease 2019—COVID-NET, 14 States, March 1–30, 2020". *MMWR* (2020) 69: 458–464. doi: 10.15585/mmwr.mm6915e3.

20 Yancy CW. "COVID-19 and African Americans". *JAMA* (2020) 323: 1891–1892. doi: 10.1001/jama.2020.6548.

21 Gomes C, McGuire TG. "Identifying the Source of Racial and Ethnic Disparities". In: Smedley B, Stith AY, Nelson AR, editors. *Unequal Treatment*. National Academies Press; Washington, DC, USA: 2003.

22 Gupta S. "Why African Americans May Be Especially Vulnerable to COVID-19" (2020). Available online: https://www.sciencenews.org/article/coronavirus-why-african-americans-vulnerable-covid-19-health-race. Accessed 28 Apr. 2020.

23 Conticini E, Frediani B, Caro D. "Can Atmospheric Pollution be Considered a Co-factor in Extremely High Level of SARS-CoV-2 Lethality in Northern Italy?" *Environ Pollut* (2020): 114465. doi: 10.1016/j.envpol.2020.114465.

24 Holmes L., Jr. *Applied Epidemiologic Principles and Concepts: Clinicians' Guide to Study Design and Conduct*. CRC Press; Boca Raton, FL, USA: 2017.

25 Hammond E. "Coronavirus Hits Black Communities Harder than Others" (2020). Available online: https://edition.cnn.com/world/live-news/coronavirus-pandemic-04–07–20/h_82cdc1a91f18f9439d6d 342de2a01f7a. Accessed 28 Apr. 2020.

26 Evelyn K. "'It's a Racial Justice Issue': Black Americans Are Dying in Greater Numbers from Covid-19". [(accessed on 2 May 2020)]; Available online: https://www.theguardian.com/world/2020/apr/08/its-a-racial-justice-issue-black-americans-are-dying-in-greater-numbers-from-covid-19. Accessed 2 May 2020.

27 Obermeyer Z, Powers B, Vogeli C, Mullainathan S. "Dissecting Racial Bias in an Algorithm Used to Manage the Health of Populations". *Science* (2019) 366: 447–453. doi: 10.1126/science.aax2342.

28 U.S. Department of Health and Human Services CDC Health Disparities and Inequalities Report: United States, 2013. *MMWR* (2013) 62: 184.

29 Penner LA, Irene V, Blair IV, Albrecht T, Dovidio JF. "Reducing Racial Health Care Disparities: A Social Psychological Analysis". *Policy Insights Behav Brain Sci* (2014) 1:204–212. doi: 10.1177/2372732214548430.

30 Subramanian SV, Acevedo-Garcia D, Osypuk TL. "Racial Residential Segregation and Geographic Heterogeneity in Black/White Disparity in Poor Self-rated Health in the US: A Multilevel Statistical Analysis". *Social Sci Med* (2005) 60: 1667–1679. doi: 10.1016/j.socscimed.2004.08.040.

31 Dorn A, Cooney R, Sabin M. "COVID-19 Exacerbating Inequalities in the US". *Lancet* (2020) 395: 1243–1244. doi: 10.1016/S0140–6736(20)30893-X.

32 Weller C. *African Americans Face Systematic Obstacles to Getting Good Jobs—Center for American Progress.* Center for American Progress; Washington, DC, USA: 2019.

33 Braveman P and Gottlieb L. "The Social Determinants of Health: It's Time to Consider the Causes of the Causes". *Public Health Rep* (2014) 129(Suppl. 2): 19–31. doi: 10.1177/00333549141291S206.

34 Rodriguez-Iturbe B and Johnson R. "Genetic Polymorphisms in Hypertension: Are We Missing the Immune Connection?" *Am J Hypertens* (2020) 32: 113–122. doi: 10.1093/ajh/hpy168.

35 Holmes L, Shutman E, Chinaka C, Deepika K, Pelaez L, Dabney KW. "Aberrant Epigenomic Modulation of Glucocorticoid Receptor Gene (NR3C1) in Early Life Stress and Major Depressive Disorder Correlation: Systematic Review and Quantitative Evidence Synthesis". *Int J Environ Res Public Health* (2019) 16: 4280. doi: 10.3390/ijerph16214280.

36 Holmes L, Lim A, Comeaux CR, Dabney KW, Okundaye O. "DNA Methylation of Candidate Genes (ACE II, IFN-γ, AGTR 1, CKG, ADD1, SCNN1B and TLR2) in Essential Hypertension: A Systematic Review and Quantitative Evidence Synthesis". *Int J Environ Res Public Health* (2019) 16: 4829. doi: 10.3390/ijerph16234829.

37 Hughes T. "Poor, Essential and on the Bus: Coronavirus is Putting Public Transportation Riders at Risk. Available online: https://www.usatoday.com/story/news/nation/2020/04/14/public-transportation-users-risk-coronavirus-spreads-across-us/2979779001/. Accesed 16 May 2020.

27 Epidemiologic Risk Modeling of Disproportionate Burden of SARS-CoV2 and COVID-19 Mortality among Racial/Ethnic Minorities (Social Class) in Washington, DC, USA

Introduction

The SARS-CoV2, causative pathogen in COVID-19, remains a pandemic, suggestive of reliable scientific control and preventive measures in flattening the epidemic curve, mitigating case fatality and mortality reduction.[1,2,3,4] The utilization of what is scientifically understood about the risk of transmission, incubation period, clinical manifestations, management, and control, is needed now more than ever before in flattening the epidemic curve both nationally and globally as well as in mortality reduction. Epidemiologic data reflects a transition from infectious disease, as the leading cause of death in the 1900s, to chronic disease in the current era, namely cardiovascular diseases (CVDs).[5,6] This scientific experience provided substantial data to epidemiology on infectious disease modeling in terms of transmission, incubation period, subclinical disease, and the period of infectivity, prognosis and fatality. Additionally, through intense screening and pathogen detection processes, epidemiologic approaches to infectious disease, as observed in the epidemic curve, could be due to excess fatality or transmission, containment and mitigation.

COVID-19, a respiratory and pulmonary disease caused by SARS-CoV2, remains a pandemic; yet, the viral dynamics, prognosis, mortality risk and subpopulation differentials in survival are not fully understood. With the onset of this condition established in the US during early March, 2020, variability in subpopulations transmission, incidence and mortality had been observed. In states with early data on socio-demographics including race, ethnicity, age and gender, disproportionate cumulative incidence (CmI) and increased case fatality had been illustrated among racial/ethnic minorities namely Blacks/African Americans (AA) and Hispanics.[7] The observed disproportionate burden in these populations has been attributed to social inequity, social gradient and social determinants of health, namely low socioeconomic status (SES), housing/living conditions, education, adverse neighborhood environment, health care access/utilization and food insecurity, as well as comorbidities.

Regarding viral spread, contact with the exposed individual, either symptomatic or asymptomatic as in SARS-CoV2, increases the transmission, which explains the rationale for increased transmission and mortality among Blacks/AA.[8] Blacks/AA reside in dense population areas with crowded housing and suffer adverse environmental neighborhood factors, such as limited green spaces, recreational facilities, safe playgrounds and transportation systems. Blacks/AA relative to their White counterparts are more likely to use public transportation systems such as transit buses, which carries a higher probability of contact with infected COVID-19 cases, increasing the risk of infectivity among Blacks/AA.[7] Since a respiratory virus such as SARS-CoV2 compromises the airways resulting in acute respiratory distress syndrome, previous exposure to environmental pollutants and toxins precipitates poor prognosis.[9,10] Such would

DOI: 10.4324/9781003424451-27

be the case in a population associated with exposure to environmental toxins and pollutants, particularly Blacks/AA.[9,10]

With evidence-based data assessment from pandemics and epidemics reflecting higher case fatality among the socially disadvantaged, such as the poor, underserved and Blacks/AA (racial minority), this study intends to examine the current experience of COVID-19 in recommending urgent equitable preparedness in addressing mortality and case fatality in the US. With structural or organized racism as the main predisposition of Blacks/AA to excess pandemic mortality, the application of the public health disproportionate universalism that mandates equitable allocation of the resources necessary for optimal health and enhanced survival, should be implemented in a timely matter. The assessment of these risk factors, such as income, SES, health insurance, safe neighborhood environment, access/utilization of quality healthcare, and lifestyles such as smoking, vaping, alcohol, drugs, and physical inactivity allow for an effective intervention mapping in addressing the disproportionate burden of this pandemic among the populations of color. These risk variables are driven by structural racism, social inequity and social gradient.

The current study aimed to assess the racial/ethnic variability in SARS-CoV2 positivity and COVID-19 mortality in the District of Columbia, Washington, DC. This predictive model examined the pre- (November, 2020) and post-thanksgiving (December, 2020) data for trends. Washington, DC, size reflects the highest population among Blacks/AA, intermediate among Whites and lowest among Hispanics, American Indians/Alaska Natives, etc.

Materials and Methods

Design

Cross-sectional ecologic design was used to assess the COVID-19 cases and mortality in the state of Washington, DC, during the last week of November and the first week of December, 2020. A novel research methodologic approach for reliable and valid evidence discovery termed Signal Application and Risk Specific Stratification (SARSS-m) model was used.[11]

Data Source and Variables Ascertainment

The aggregate data utilized in this assessment were from the Washington DC Department of Health (https://coronavirus.dc.gov/data). To assess trends and the direction as either positive or negative in pattern, data from the last week in November and the first week in December 2020 were examined. Washington DC Department of Health. The variables examined were confirmed or positive cases, deaths, age, gender, race/ethnicity and wards as geographic, zip codes and county. The US Census data 2020 were used to determine the population size of Washington, DC, by race/ethnicity prior to the computation of the disproportionate burden of SARS-CoV2 case positivity and mortality.

Statistical Analyses

The fatality proportion was estimated using the number of death/confirmed cases, multiplied by 100 (Fatality Percentage (%) or proportion). Line graphs and the linear model with the coefficient of determination (R^2) were used to illustrate the case fatalities and transmission. While chi square statistic (X^2) was used to test independence by race/ethnicity. The binomial regression model was utilized for risk stratification modeling, but could not address and control for the confounding due to limited data on social determinants of health and population health dynamics.

Case Fatality Modeling

To determine the daily percent change (DPC) in case fatality modeling for upward (positive) or downward (negative) trend, we utilized the formula D2-D1/D1*100, implying case fatality in the end result or End Result Case Fatality (ERCF) or (D2) – Baseline Case Fatality (BCF)*100. Therefore, DPC = ERCF-BCF/BCF*100.[11]

The type I error tolerance was set at 0.05 (95% CI) and all tests were two tailed. The entire analyses were performed using STATA, Version 16.0 (StataCorp., College Station, TX, USA).

Results

These data represent the SARS-CoV2 case positivity and COVID-19 mortality by race/ethnicity, sex, ward as geographic locale and age. With the study focus being race/ethnicity, patterns with respect to temporal trends, comparing the last week in November and the first week in December 2020 were examined, indicative of a positive trend in SARS-CoV2 positivity and COVID-19 mortality during this period. Similarly, COVID-19 mortality illustrated a positive across all race/ethic groups, especially among Blacks/AA.

SARS-CoV2 Case Positivity and COVID-19 Morality Cumulative Incidence (CmI) by Race/ethnicity, Sex, Age and Geographic Locale (Ward)

Although not in the tables, during late November 2020, the SARS-CoV2 case positivity in Washington, DC, was higher among Blacks/AA (*n* = 9,441 (46.7%) relative to Whites, 4,603 (22.8%). With respect to Hispanics, the SARS-CoV2 case positivity was 4,853 (24.1%) and 13,477 (66.9%) among non-Hispanics. Regarding COVID-19 mortality, this was lowest among non-Hispanic Whites (NHW), 1.50%, intermediate among Hispanics (1.81%), and highest among non-Hispanic Blacks (NHB), 5.30%. Regardless of temporality, there was a sex differential in mortality cumulative incidence (CmI), with males (57.0%) compared to females (43.0%) illustrating higher mortality. The mortality CmI by age was lowest among cases, 20–29 years (6.4%), intermediate among cases, 50–69 years (36.3%) and highest among individuals, 70 years and older (58.7%). With respect to the geographic locale (DC-Ward), the mortality CmI was higher in wards DC-4–6 (39.3%) and wards DC-7–8 (35.4%) but lower in wards DC-1–3 (22.1%). During the first week in December, post-thanksgiving period, the

Table 27.1 SARS-Cov-2 Case Positivity by Race/Ethnicity, December 2020, Washington, DC

Variable	SARS-Cov-2 Case Positivity, December 2020					
Race/Ethnicity	3-Dec	4-Dec	5-Dec	6-Dec	7-Dec	8-Dec
	n (%)	n (%)	n (%)	n (%)	n (%)	n (%)
White (NHW)	5,311 (23.6)	5,426 (23.7)	5,531 (23.9)	5,589 (24)	5,653 (24.1)	5,719 (24.3)
Black (NHB)	10,353 (46.7)	10,670 (46.7)	10,846 (46.9)	10,951 (47)	11,077 (47.1)	11,218 (47)
Hispanic	5,241 (23.3)	5,313 (23.3)	5,364 (23.2)	5,420 (23.3)	5,473 (23.2)	5,515 (23.1)

Notes, abbreviations and Data Source: The SARS-CoV2 case positivity percentage or proportion was estimated using all those who were tested for SARS-CoV2 the COVID-19 causing pathogen divided by the total number of those tested positive. *n* = number or frequency, % = percentage, Dec = December, NHW = Non-Hispanic White, NHB = Non-Hispanic Blacks.
Data Source: Washington DC Department of Health, USA.

SARS-Cov-2 case positivity was lower among Whites (*n*, 5,719, (23.0%)) compared to Blacks/ AA, 11,218 (47%).

Figure 27.1 illustrates SARS-CoV2 case positivity by race/ethnicity during November, 2020. This linear graph presents NHB with the highest case fatality while Hispanics and NHW indicated intermediate and lowest case fatality, respectively. Similarly, Figure 27.2 exhibits case fatality by race/ethnicity during December 2020 with highest case fatality observed among NHB, and was intermediate among Hispanics but lowest among NHW.

SARS-CoV2 Case Positivity by Race/Ethnicity

Table 27.1 illustrates SARS-CoV2 positivity stratified by race/ethnicity between December 3 and 8, 2021 in Washington, DC. Despite the observed SARS-CoV2 confirmed cases, which plateaued during this period among Hispanics, marginal positive trends were observed among Blacks/AA and Whites. The SARS-CoV2 CmI was higher among Blacks/AA relative to Whites, as well as higher among non-Hispanics compared to their Hispanic counterparts. Concerning the burden of SARS-CoV2 case positivity in Washington, DC, Blacks/AA and Hispanics were observed with the disproportionate burden SARS-CoV2 transmission and infectivity.

COVID-19 Mortality by Race/Ethnicity

Table 27.2 demonstrates the COVID-19 mortality CmI by race/ethnicity during the first week in December 2020 in Washington, DC. The CmI for NHW ranged from 10.0% to 10.3%, while the range for NHB was 74.0% to 74.2%, and ranged from 13.2% to 13.3%. The COVID-19

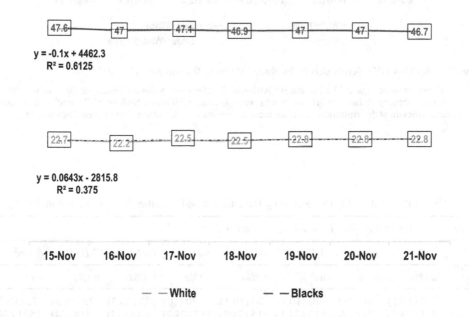

Figure 27.1 SARS-CoV2 Seropositivity, Washington, DC, November, 2020

Notes and abbreviations: Figure 27.1 illustrates SARS-CoV2 seropositivity during November 2020 in Washington, DC, USA by race. Relative to Whites, Blacks were observed with higher SARS-CoV2 cumulative incidence. The R^2 is the coefficient of determination, implying the Y determinant as X, independent or predictor variable. Nov = November R^2 = Coefficient of determination Y = SARS-CoV2 seropositive, and X = time trends as independent or predictor variable in linear estimate, while Y is the outcome variable.

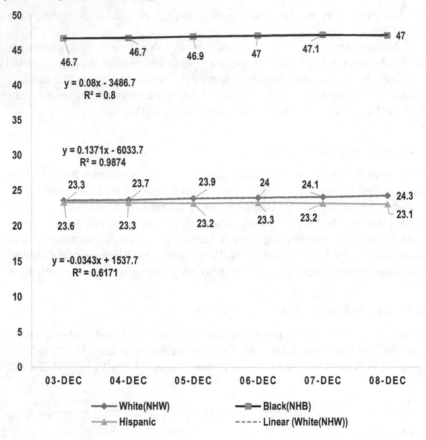

Figure 27.2 SARS-COV2 Seropositivity by Race/Ethnicity, Washington, DC, 2020

Notes and abbreviations: Figure 27.2 illustrates SARS-CoV2 seropositivity during December 2020 in Washington, DC, USA by race/ethnicity. Relative to Whites, Blacks were observed with higher SARS-CoV2 cumulative incidence. The R^2 is the coefficient of determination, implying the Y determinant as X, independent or predictor variable.

Table 27.2 COVID-19 Mortality Prevalence by Race/Ethnicity, December 2020, Washington, DC

Variable	COVID-19 Mortality Prevalence, December 2020							
Race/ Ethnicity	1-Dec	2-Dec	3-Dec	4-Dec	5-Dec	6-Dec	7-Dec	8-Dec
	n (%)	n (%)	n (%)	n (%)	n (%)	n (%)	n (%)	n (%)
NHW	70 (10.1)	70 (10.1)	70 (10.1)	70 (10.1)	70 (10)	72 (10.3)	72 (10.3)	72 (10.2)
NHB	511 (74.1)	512 (74)	513 (74.1)	515 (74.1)	517 (74.2)	518 (74)	518 (74)	521 (74)
Hispanic	91 (13.2)	92 (13.3)	92 (13.3)	92 (13.3)	92 (13.2)	93 (13.3)	93 (13.3)	93 (13.2)

Notes, abbreviations and Data Source: The mortality prevalence as cumulative mortality was estimated using sub-population mortality divided by the total daily mortality. *n* = number or frequency, % = percentage, Dec = December, NHW = Non-Hispanic White, NHB = Non-Hispanic Blacks.
Data Source: Washington DC Department of Health, USA.

CmI mortality was highest among Blacks/AA as NHB, intermediate among Hispanics and lowest among Whites as NHW. Racial/ethnic minorities demonstrate the disproportionate burden of COVID-19 based on population size. The CmI mortality was highest among NHB, $n =$ 521 (74%), intermediate among Hispanics, $n = 93$ (13.2%) and lowest among NHW, $n = 72$, (10.2%). While Blacks represent an estimated 48% to 49% of the Washington, DC, population, the COVID-19 mortality was 74% among them, indicative of the disproportionate burden of COVID-19 mortality. In the same vein, while Hispanics account for 8.8% of the Washington, DC, population, COVID-19 mortality among them was 13.0%, indicative of excess mortality in this minority population. Figure 27.3 presents COVID-19 CmI by race/ethnicity during December 2020. There were racial/ethnic mortality differentials, with the highest mortality CmI observed among Blacks/AA, while intermediate and lowest mortality CmI were observed among Hispanics and Whites, respectively.

COVID-19 Case Fatality Proportion, Stratified by Race/Ethnicity

Table 27.3 exhibits COVID-19 case fatality in Washington, DC, during December 2020, stratified by race/ethnicity. Commencing December 1 to December 8, 2020, there were racial/ethnic

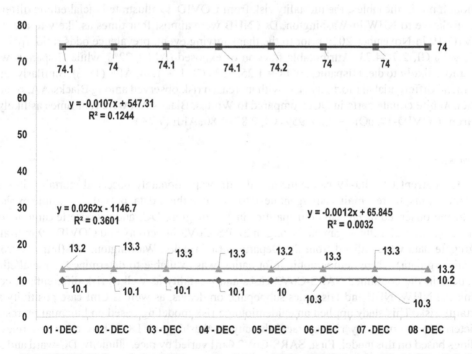

Figure 27.3 COVID-19 Cumulative Incidence (CmI) Mortality by Race/Ethnicity, Washington DC, 2020

Notes, abbreviations and Data Source: Figure 27.3 illustrates SARS-CoV2 seropositivity during December, 2020 in Washington, DC, USA by race/ethnicity. Relative to Whites, Blacks were observed with higher SARS-CoV2 cumulative incidence. The R^2 is the coefficient of determination, implying the Y determinant as X, independent or predictor variable. Dec = December, NHW = Non-Hispanic White, NHB = Non-Hispanic Blacks.

Data Source: Washington DC Department of Health, USA.

Table 27.3 COVID-19 Case Fatality Proportion by Race/Ethnicity, December 2020, Washington, DC

Variable	COVID-19 Case Fatality, December 2020							
Race/ ethnicity	1-Dec	2-Dec	3-Dec	4-Dec	5-Dec	6-Dec	7-Dec	8-Dec
	%	%	%	%	%	%	%	%
NHW	1.35	1.33	1.32	1.3	1.27	1.29	1.29	1.26
NHB	5	4.95	4.9	4.81	4.8	4.73	4.68	4.64
Hispanic	1.76	1.77	1.76	1.73	1.72	1.72	1.71	1.69

Notes, abbreviations and Data Source: The case fatality proportion or prevalence was estimated using the total mortality in a specific subpopulation divided by the total case positivity in that subpopulation. % = percentage, Dec = December, NHW = Non-Hispanic White, NHB = Non-Hispanic Blacks.
Data Source: Washington DC Department of Health, USA.

differentials in case fatality. The case fatality proportion was highest among NHB, ranging from 4.64% to 5.00%, intermediate among Hispanics, ranging from 1.69% to 1.73%, and lowest among NHW, 1.26% to 1.35%. The case fatality was highest among NHB, intermediate among Hispanics but lowest among NHW.

COVID-19 Mortality Risk Model

Although not in the tables, the mortality risk from COVID-19 illustrated racial/ethnic differentials. Relative to NHW in Washington, DC, NHB were almost four times as likely to die from COVID-19 in November 2020 prior to the thanksgiving event, prevalence odds ratio, (pOR) = 3.62, 95% CI, 2.78-4.73. Attributable fraction of exposed (AFE), 72%, while Hispanics were 25% more likely to die, Hispanics, pOR = 1.25, 95% CI, 1.0–1.74, AFE (18%). Similarly, there was racial differential in mortality risk, with increased risk observed among Blacks/AA, relative to their White counterparts in DC. Compared to Whites, Blacks/AA were four times as likely to die from COVID-19, pOR = 4.00, 95% CI, 2.87–4.80, AFE (73%).

Discussion

With the current COVID-19 pandemic and the disproportionately observed mortality in some subpopulations, there remains an urgent need to examine these data, provide a possible explanation to the observed racial /ethnic disparities in Washington, DC, and propose feasible recommendations in racial/ethnic gap narrowing in SARS-CoV2 infectivity and COVID-19 mortality. Aggregate data were utilized from the Department of Health, Washington, DC (https://coronavirus.dc.org/data) where demographic information was available to determine the racial/ethnic variances in the confirmed SARS-CoV2 cases and mortality as well as risk differentials, comparing the NHW, NHB and Hispanics subpopulation deaths, as well as CmI case positivity and mortality risk. This study applied an epidemiologic risk modeling based on binomial regression to determine the mortality risk by race/ethnicity in Washington, DC. There are a few relevant findings based on this model. First, SARS-CoV2 CmI varied by race, ethnicity, DC-ward and sex. Second, there was a disproportionate burden of COVID-19 mortality among NHB and Hispanics. Third, the case fatality was higher among NHB relative to NHW. Fourthly, NHB relative to NHW regardless of DC-ward presented with excess mortality and increased COVID-19 mortality risk.

We have demonstrated that SARS-CoV2 CmI varied by race, ethnicity, DC-ward and sex. The CmI was highest among NHW, intermediate among NHB and Hispanics, but lowest among

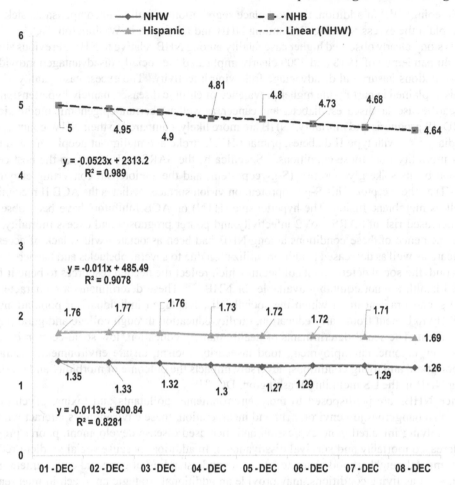

Figure 27.4 COVID-19 Case Fatality by Race/Ethnicity, Washington, DC, December, 2020

Notes and abbreviations: Dec = December, NHB = Non-Hispanic Blacks, NHW = Non-Hispanic Whites, R^2 = Coefficient of determination, Y = SARS-CoV2 seropositive, and X = time trends as independent or predictor variable.

Asian/Pacific Islanders. However, NHB and Hispanics illustrated the disproportionate burden of SARS-CoV2. Previous literature had observed a comparable pattern of transmission in different settings[7]. The observed burden of SARS-CoV2 CmI among NHB is explained by workplace segregation, where NHB are employed in jobs with fewer or no benefits, but with more adverse conditions, such as buildings with no fire exit,[12] as well as a stressful environment in Washington, DC. Specifically, NHB and Hispanics who are employed as public transit drivers have an increased risk of contracting viral microbes, which also explains the COVID-19 racial and ethnic burden differentials.

The current has also observed an increased SARS-CoV2 disproportionate burden of CmI among residents in some DC-wards as well as disproportionate burden between NHB and Hispanics in these wards. The observed COVID-19 mortality differences by DC-ward is due to the increasing population density of NHB and Hispanics in these wards, as well as the type of employment which predisposed these subpopulations to increased exposure to environments with exponential viral spread such as, sanitation job, maids, and restaurant and hotels housekeeping.[13,14,15] In addition, the workplace segregation as well as uncompensated sick time may explain the excess SARS-CoV2 among NHB and Hispanics in Washington, DC.

This study clearly observed higher case fatality among NHB relative to NHW. Previous studies in the flu pandemics of 1918 and 2009 clearly implicated the socially disadvantaged individuals and populations in survival disadvantage following infectivity.[7] The excess case fatality among NHB is explained in part by the higher prevalence of chronic diseases, namely hypertension and other cardiovascular diseases, diabetes and cancer, as well as aberrant epigenomic modulation in COVID-19 prognosis and mortality.[7] NHB are more likely, compared to their NHW counterparts, to be diagnosed with type II diabetes, primary HTN, stroke and malignant neoplasm[16] and have higher mortality from these conditions.[17] Specifically, the SARS-CoV2 entry to the host cell is mediated by its spike glycoprotein (S-glycoprotein) and the angiotensin converting enzyme II (ACE-II) as the receptor. This S-glycoprotein on virion surface mediates the ACE II recognition as well as membrane fusion. The hypertensive (HTN) on ACE Inhibitors have been observed with increased risk of SARS-CoV2 infectivity and poorer prognoses and excess mortality. The higher incidence of these conditions among NHB had been associated with a lack of access to healthcare as well as decreased healthcare utilization due to several obstacles and barriers.[17]

Second, the social determinants of health which reflect the needed resources to benefit from optimal health are not equitably available for NHB.[17,18] These determinants are characterized by the social gradient upon which the socially disadvantaged individuals or populations are less likely to benefit from early education, quality education through college and good paying employment. The social determinants of health, namely education, low socio-economic status (SES), low income, unemployment, food insecurity, racism, unsafe environment, insurance, transportation, and living conditions, adversely impacts the outcome of morbidity and mortality among NHB in the US including Washington, DC.[19,20,21]

Since NHBs are predisposed to more environmental pollutants and toxins, psychosocial stressors, a dangerous job environment and incarceration, these environments interact with the gene, implying impaired gene expression and increased disease development, poorer prognosis, increased mortality and survival disadvantage. In addition, because social gradient reflects environmental neighborhood characteristics, the understanding of gene and environment interaction, such as living conditions, may provide an additional strategic approach in intervention mapping for disease management and prevention. In effect, examining the gene and environment interaction, observed as epigenomic modulations, will provide substantial data on intervention mapping in narrowing the gaps between NHB and NHW in Washington, DC, with respect to COVID-19 mortality.

The gene and environment interaction as epigenomic modulations that commence at gametogenesis are transgenerational but reversible. The social signal transduction that is evoked from the stress placed on NHB and Hispanics has a substantial effect on the sympathetic nervous system, provoking the beta-adrenergic receptors. This response has been shown to involve the Conserved Transcriptional Response to Adversity (CTRA) gene expression and the consequent elaboration of pro-inflammatory cytokines, due to the impaired gene expression of the transcription factors (transcriptomes) and the inhibition of gene expression with respect to anti-inflammatory response.[22] In understanding these pathways of genomic stability and their role in disease causation as well as mortality, epigenomic studies are necessary in determining whether or not Blacks/AA, relative to Whites, have an increased mean deoxyribonucleic acid (DNA) methylation index with respect to the genome-wide analysis. Such initiative will involve the utilization of the bisulfite pyrosequencing that is very specific in differentiating between the methyl group (CH_3) and hydroxymethyl group, as well as the binding of these groups to the Cytosine-phosphate-Guanine (CpG) region of the gene, inhibiting transcription and the messenger ribonucleic acid (mRNA) sequencing, leading to impaired gene expression and abnormal cellular functionality. The reference to epigenomics investigation reflects the inability of a COVID-19 case to respond to treatment modalities due to the drug receptors unavailability, resulting from impaired gene expression (mRNA translation dysregulation) reflecting decreased response to COVID-19 treatment among racial/ethnic minorities namely NHB and Hispanics.[21] The observed epigenomic aberration clearly illustrates treatment effect heterogeneity in which some subpopulations respond differentially to a given therapeutic agent in the phase of epigenomic lesion, explaining in part racial risk differentials in COVID-19 case fatality. Further, if DNA hypermethylation facilitates the host cell SARS-CoV2 spike glycoprotein binding to ACE-II as well as the membrane fusion, therefore subpopulations with aberrant epigenomic modulations characterized by DNA hypermethylation.

Despite the rigorous methodology utilized in this racial/ethnic mortality risk model for SARS-CoV2 and COVID-19, there are some limitations. First this study utilized pre-existing data as secondary data as ecologic (aggregate, not individual level) which are subject to information, selection and misclassification biases. However, the observed disproportionate burden of SARS-CoV2 CmI among NHB and Hispanics in Washington, DC, is not driven solely by these biases. Second, since risks do not occur in isolation, requiring an application of explanatory model, namely confounding adjustment, it is unlikely that the predictive mortality risk in this study which implicated increased COVID-19 mortality and case fatality among NHB and Hispanics is driven solely by these unmeasured confounders.[23]

Conclusions and Recommendations

Washington, DC, SARS-CoV2 case positivity, case fatality and mortality risk indicate a disproportionate burden of COVID-19 on the communities of color, namely NHB and Hispanics. In addition, there was a positive trend in SARS-CoV2 transmission as well as comparable case fatality and mortality risk characterization by race/ethnicity. These findings are indicative of the need to examine subpopulations health and social needs, namely NHB and Hispanics for intervention mapping for SARS-CoV2 transmission reduction, racial/ethnic case fatality and mortality gap narrowing. The epidemiologic perspective in control and prevention recommends:

(1) An urgent and increasing need for adherence to preventive and control measures in these subpopulations at risk for transmission reduction, mainly Hispanics and NHB, including testing, contact tracing, tracking, social and physical distancing as well as non-surgical and non-medical face mask utilization while outside home.
(2) Further, these findings are suggestive of the need to examine the social gradient that may be associated with the disproportionate burden of mortality among NHB and Hispanics as well as an explanation for the increased risk of transmission among Hispanics and NHB in DC-wards. (a) The application of these recommendations will enhance Washington, DC, in curve flattening and down drifting as well as case fatality mitigation especially among the marginalized and most vulnerable populations, namely NHB, American Indian/Alaska Natives and Hispanics. (b) Since health equity is essential in subpopulations risk and health outcomes marginalization, this study clearly recommends Washington, DC, to utilize disproportionate benefit for NHB and Hispanics for equitable outcome of SARS-CoV2 transmission and COVID-19 case fatality and mortality.
(3) Social and physical distancing until the epidemic curve is flattened in Washington, DC, prior to the return to a normal economic life, will prevent a significant resurgence of COVID-19 with altered SARS-CoV2 antigenicity or different serotypes.

(4) Facemask application throughout the state, especially among COVID-19 positives and symptomatic individuals to marginalize the spread of the virus.

(5) The immune system potentiation by providing equitable resources to Blacks/AA and Hispanics who are socially disadvantaged with low SES in Washington, DC. In addition, since history is relevant to human health and survival, we must continue to maintain appointment with history. However, history of the Tuskegee Syphilis Experiment of the 1930s should not determine our destiny on SARS-CoV2 vaccination.

(6) The education of the NHB and Hispanic communities on the health consequences of COVID-19 through ePublic Health Intervention program and the provision of assistance and encouragement for testing, case identification and isolation will flatten the epidemic curve in the Black/AA communities. This initiative will not only reduce social inequities but also the social inequities burden for future disease and pandemics.

(7) Since the disproportionate burden of pandemics fundamentally reflects health disparities, addressing this disproportionate burden in future epidemics and pandemics will require subpopulations, especially NHB, American Indians/Alaska Native and Hispanics to be provided with the resources necessary for optimal health. Therefore, adherence to the World Health Organization's recommendation of social justice and peace as conditions necessary for health is essential in narrowing health disparities in pandemics by addressing now social injustice and systemic and structural racism, thus transforming health equity. Washington, DC, through the Center for Disease Control and Prevention (CDC), is to increase testing throughout DC, especially in the most vulnerable COVID-19 population, namely NHB and Hispanics.

(8) The development of surveillance and monitoring systems for data availability on the social determinants of health and race/ethnicity in transforming pandemic health equity is essential in intervention mapping in marginalizing the COVID-19 outcomes among the communities of color.

(9) Establishment and implementation of a rapid health equity transformation taskforce and evaluation matrix for risk mitigation among racial and ethnic minorities, namely Blacks/AA and Hispanics.

(10) As the mRNA vaccine for SARS-CoV2 host "spike" protein generation for antibody production, the administration of this novel technology vaccine must be widely available among the most vulnerable populations, especially the socially disadvantaged population, namely NHB and Hispanics for herd immunity in these subpopulations prior to other communities' immunizations in Washington, DC.

With these data on racial/ethnic differentials in COVID-19 mortality risk, as emergency preparedness, health equity resources are required through disproportionate universalism, which is the public health lens in the provision of health services more to the racial/ethnic minorities prior to the non-vulnerable populations. The failure to address the socially disadvantaged individuals and populations' needs in our society, namely Washington, DC, by educational opportunity, equitable employment opportunity and the departure from structural racism, will render the NHB and Hispanics in DC more vulnerable to public health and healthcare crises in this pandemic and the current surge with the new SARS-CoV2 variants. In effect, as clinicians, researchers, health officers, epidemiologist, infectious disease specialist and public health experts, it is our moral responsibility regardless of our race/ethnicity, gender or age, to rapidly respond to the disproportionate mortality burden of this pandemic in the communities of color, especially NHB and Hispanics, since human life remains a primary value.

Questions for Discussion

1. What is the research question and hypothesis utilized in this analytic epidemiologic study on SARS-CoV2 and COVID-19?
2. Describe the epidemiologic design utilized in this study and examine the data source.
3. Is this study a primary or secondary data assessment in SARS-CoV2 seropositivity and COVID-19 mortality?
4. What is the statistical analytic method utilized in these data assessment?
5. Are these data ecologic or individual level data? What are the limitations in the utilization of an ecologic data in SARS-CoV2 seropositivity and COVID-19 mortality parameter estimation?
6. What are the main findings in this study and the limitations of this study?
7. Is there confounding assessment in this study, and the inclusion of such variables in a reliable parameter estimate, with respect to the nexus between the independent and outcome variable? Was the effect measure modifier as heterogeneity effect observed in this study?
8. Is the inference or conclusion reliable and accurate?
9. What are the suggestions or recommendation in future research?
10. Are the references appropriately cited?

Notes

1 Anderson RM, Heesterbeek H, Klinkenberg D, Hollingsworth TD. "How Will Country-based Mitigation Measures Influence the Course of the COVID-19 Epidemic?" *Lancet* (2020) 395(10228): 931 934. https://doi.org/10.1016/S0140–6736(20)30567-5.

2 Giwa A, Desai A, Duca A. (2020). "Novel 2019 Coronavirus SARS-CoV-2 (COVID-19): An Overview for Emergency Clinicians". *Emerg Med Pract* (2020) 22(2 Suppl 2): 1–28.

3 Estreicher M, Hranjec T, Pepe PE et al. "Spotting the Clotting: Hypercoagulopathy in COVID-19". (2020). Available at: https://www.emsworld.com/1224381/spotting-clotting-hypercoagulopathy-covid-19. Accessed 20 Nov. 2020.

4 Bikdeli B, Madhavan MV, Jimenez D, Chuich T, Dreyfus I, Driggin E, et al. (2020). "COVID-19 and Thrombotic or Thromboembolic Disease: Implications for Prevention, Antithrombotic Therapy, and Follow-up". *J Am Coll Cardiol* (2020) 75(23) [epub ahead of print]. doi:10.1016/j.jacc.2020.04.031.

5 Omran AR. "The Epidemiologic Transition: A Theory of the Epidemiology of Population Change. 1971". *The Milbank Quarterly* (2005) 83(4): 731–757. https://doi.org/10.1111/j.1468–0009.2005.00398.

6 McKeown RE. "The Epidemiologic Transition: Changing Patterns of Mortality and Population Dynamics". *American Journal of Lifestyle Medicine* (2009) 3(1 Suppl): 19S 26S. https://doi.org/10.1177/1559827609335350.

7 Holmes Jr, L, Enwere E, Williams J, Ogundele B, Chavan P, Piccoli T, Chinaka C, Comeaux C, Pelaez L, Okundaye O, Stalnaker L, Kalle F, Deepika K, Philipcien G, Poleon M, Ogungbade G, Elmi H, John V, Dabney KW. (2020). "Black–White Risk Differentials in COVID-19 (SARS-CoV-2) Transmission, Mortality and Case Fatality in the United States: Translational Epidemiologic Perspective and Challenges". *Int J Environ Res Public Health* (2020) 17(2): 4322. doi:10.3390/ijerph17124322.

8 Rothe C, Schunk M, Sothmann P, et al. "Transmission of 2019-nCoV Infection from an Asymptomatic Contact in Germany". *N Engl J Med* (2020) 382(10): 970–971. doi:10.1056/NEJMc2001468.

9 Singhal T. (2020). "A Review of Coronavirus Disease-2019 (COVID-19)". *Indian Journal of Pediatrics* (2020) 87(4): 281–286. https://doi.org/10.1007/s12098-020-03263-6.

10 Holmes Jr, L. "Applied Epidemiologic Principles and Concept: Clinician's Guidelines to Study Conduct and Interpretation, CRC". (2018). Available at: https://www.routledge.com/Applied-Epidemiologic-Principles-and-Concepts-Clinicians-Guide-to-Study/Jr/p/book/9780367560089. Accessed 18 Nov. 2020.

11 Mohanty SK, Satapathy A, Naidu MM, Mukhopadhyay S, Sharma S, Barton LM, Stroberg E, Duval EJ, Pradhan D, Tzankov A, Parwani AV. "Severe Acute Respiratory Syndrome Coronavirus-2 (SARS-CoV-2) and Coronavirus Disease 19 (COVID-19) – Anatomic Pathology Perspective on Current Knowledge". *Diagnostic Pathology* (2020) 15(1): 103. https://doi.org/10.1186/s13000-020-01017-8.

12 DHSS, Delaware Health and Social Services. "My Healthy Community: Delaware Environmental Public Health Tracking Network". Available at: https://myhealthycommunity.dhss.delaware.gov/locations/state. Accessed 21 Nov. 2020.

13 Gee, GC and Ford CL. "Structural Racism and Health Inequities: Old Issues, New Directions". *Du Bois Review: Social Science Research on Race* (2011) 8(1): 115–132. https://doi.org/10.1017/S1742058X11000130.

14 Krogstad JM, Gonzalez-Barrera A, Lopez MH. "Hispanics more likely than Americans overall to see coronavirus as a major threat to health and finances". Pew Research Center (2020). Available at: https://www.pewresearch.org/fact-tank/2020/03/24/hispanics-more-likely-than-americans-overall-to-see-coronavirus-as-a-major-threat-to-health-and-finances/. Accessed 20 Nov. 2020.

15 Despres C. "Coronavirus Case Rates and Death Rates for Latinos in the United States. Salud America!" (2020). Available at: https://salud-america.org/coronavirus-case-rates-and-death-rates-for-latinos-in-the-united-states/. Accessed 20 Nov. 2020.

16 CDC, Centers for Disease Control and Prevention. "National Center for Health Statistics. Weekly Updates by Select Demographic and Geographic Characteristics. Provisional Death Counts for Coronavirus Disease (COVID-19)". (2020). Available at: https://www.cdc.gov/nchs/nvss/vsrr/covid_weekly/. Accessed Nov. 22, 2020.

17 Lincoln KD, Abdou CM, Lloyd D. "Race and Socioeconomic Differences in Obesity and Depression among Black and non-Hispanic White Americans". *Journal of Health Care for the Poor and Underserved* (2014) 25(1): 257–275. https://doi.org/10.1353/hpu.2014.0038.

18 Singh, GK, Daus GP, Allender M, Ramey CT, Martin E.K, Perry C, Reyes A, Vedamuthu IP. (2017). "Social Determinants of Health in the United States: Addressing Major Health Inequality Trends for the Nation, 1935–2016". *International Journal of MCH and AIDS* (2017) 6(2): 139–164. https://doi.org/10.21106/ijma.236.

19 Walker RJ, Strom Williams J, Egede LE. "Influence of Race, Ethnicity and Social Determinants of Health on Diabetes Outcomes". *The American Journal of the Medical Sciences* (2016) 351(4): 366–373. https://doi.org/10.1016/j.amjms.2016.01.008.

20 Noonan AS, Velasco-Mondragon HE, Wagner FA. "Improving the Health of African Americans in the USA: An Overdue Opportunity for Social Justice". *Public Health Rev* (2016) 37: 12. https://doi.org/10.1186/s40985-016-0025-4.

21 Holmes L Jr, Shutman E, Chinaka C, Deepika K, Pelaez L, Dabney KW. (2019). "Aberrant Epigenomic Modulation of Glucocorticoid Receptor Gene (NR3C1) in Early Life Stress and Major Depressive Disorder Correlation: Systematic Review and Quantitative Evidence Synthesis". *International Journal of Environmental Research and Public Health* (2019) 16(21): 4280. https://doi.org/10.3390/ijerph16214280.

22 Sanders JM, Monogue ML, Jodlowski TZ, Cutrell JB et al. "Pharmacologic Treatments for Coronavirus Disease 2019 (COVID-19): A Review". *JAMA* (2020) 323(18): 1824–1836. doi:10.1001/jama.2020.6019.

23 Holmes L, Chan W, Jiang Z et al. (2007). "Effectiveness of Androgen Deprivation Therapy in Prolonging Survival of Older Men Treated for Locoregional Prostate Cancer". *Prostate Cancer Prostatic Dis* (2007) 10: 388–395. https://doi.org/10.1038/sj.pcan.4500973.

28 Racial/Ethnic and Geo-Clustering Differentials in SARS-CoV2 (COVID-19) Cumulative Incidence, Mortality and Temporal Trend in Delaware State, USA

Introduction

SARS-CoV2, causative pathogen in COVID-19, remains a global pandemic, suggestive of reliable scientific control and preventive measure response in flattening the epidemic curve and mitigating case fatality.[1,2,3,4] The utilization of what is scientifically understood about the risk of transmission, incubation period, clinical manifestations, management and control, is needed now more than ever before in flattening the epidemic curve both nationally and globally. Epidemiologic data reflects a transition from infectious disease as the leading cause of death in the 1900s to chronic disease, namely cardiovascular diseases (CVDs) in the current era.[5,6] This scientific experience provided substantial data to epidemiology on infectious disease modeling in terms of transmission, incubation period, subclinical disease, and the period of infectivity, prognosis and fatality. Additionally, epidemiologic approaches to infectious disease observed in the epidemic curve, which could be due to excess fatality or transmission containment and mitigation through intense screening and pathogen detection.

COVID-19, a respiratory and pulmonary disease caused by the SARS-CoV2 virus, remains a pandemic and not fully understood with respect to viral dynamics, prognosis, mortality risk and subpopulation differentials in survival. With the onset of this condition established in the US during early March 2020, variability in subpopulations transmission, incidence and mortality has been observed. In states with early data on socio-demographics including race, ethnicity, age and gender, disproportionate cumulative incidence (CmI) and increased case fatality has been illustrated among racial/ethnic minorities, namely Blacks/African Americans and Hispanics.[7] The observed disproportionate burden in these populations has been attributed to social inequity and social determinants of health, namely low SES, housing/living conditions, education, adverse neighborhood environment, health care access/utilization and food insecurity, as well as comorbidities.

Regarding viral spread, contact with the exposed individual, either symptomatic or asymptomatic as in SARS-CoV2 increases the transmission, which explains the rationale for increased transmission and mortality among Blacks/AA.[8] Blacks/AA reside in densely populated areas with crowded housing and suffer adverse environmental neighborhood factors, such as limited green spaces, recreational facilities, safe playgrounds and transportation systems. Blacks/AA relative to their White counterparts are more likely to use public transportation systems such as transit buses, which carries a higher probability of contact with infected COVID-19 cases, increasing the risk of infectivity among Blacks/AA.[7] Since a respiratory virus such as SARS-CoV2 compromises the airways resulting in acute respiratory distress syndrome, previous exposure to environmental pollutants and toxins precipitates poor prognosis.[9,10] However, populations associated with exposure to environmental toxins and pollutants, such as Blacks/AA, Hispanics and underserved Whites are more likely exposed to SARS-CoV2 transmission and COVID-19 case fatality and mortality.

DOI: 10.4324/9781003424451-28

With evidence-based data assessment from pandemics and epidemics, reflecting higher case fatality among the socially disadvantaged, such as the poor, underserved and Blacks/AA (racial minority), this study intends to examine the current experience of COVID-19 in recommending urgent equitable preparedness in addressing mortality and case fatality in Delaware. With structural or organized racism as the main predisposition of Blacks/AA to excess pandemic mortality, the application of the public health disproportionate universalism that mandates equitable allocation of resources necessary for optimal health and enhanced survival should be urgently implemented. The assessment of these variables such as income, SES, health insurance, safe neighborhood environment, access and utilization of quality healthcare, and lifestyles such as smoking, vaping, alcohol, drugs, physical inactivity, which are implicitly driven by structural racism, allow for an effective intervention mapping in addressing what is "avoidable" and "unacceptable", social inequity as an exposure function of health inequities and disparities in morbidity and mortality.

The current study aimed to assess the racial/ethnic and geo-clustering of COVID-19 confirmed cases and mortality in the state of Delaware, USA. We postulated that the population with disproportionate burden of diseases in the US and in all states including DE will be disproportionately affected, as well as geo-clustering of populations with disproportionate burden of socioeconomics as a social gradient such as Sussex County in DE.

Materials and Methods

Design

A cross-sectional ecologic design was used to assess COVID-19 cases and mortality in the state of DE during the last week of April and the first week of May 2020 as well as the mid-week in November for trends and patterns assessment. A novel research methodologic approach for reliable and valid evidence discovery termed Signal Application and Risk Specific Stratification (SARSS-m) model was used.[11] This model allows for sampling from a sample, given "big data", noise elimination from the data by assessing for missing variables, outliers, biologic/clinical relevance, confounding and effect measure modification prior to model specification and building.

Data Source

The aggregate data utilized in this assessment were from the Delaware Department of Health and Social Services.[12] To assess trends and the direction as either positive or negative in pattern, data collected during 14 through 20 November, 2020, were used for the case positivity, while the case fatality and mortality utilized the cumulative incidence data between 7 and 13 November 2020.

Variables Ascertainment

The variables examined were confirmed or positive cases, deaths, age, gender, race/ethnicity, zip codes and county. The US Census data 2020 were used to determine the population size of DE by race, ethnicity and sex prior to the computation of the disproportionate burden of SARS-CoV2 case positivity and COVID-19 case fatality and mortality.

Statistical Analyses

The pre-analysis screening was performed for missing data and outliers. We estimated the fatality proportion using the number of death/confirmed cases, multiplied by 100 (Fatality Percentage

(%) or proportion). The line graphs, as linear visual models, were used to illustrate case fatalities and transmission with temporal trends.

The assessment of geo-clustering of mortality and transmission was performed with a Poisson regression model. This model utilized DE as the reference and estimated the parameters for the observed zip codes in New Castle, Kent and Sussex counties. The type I error tolerance was set at 0.05 (5%) while the parameter's precision was determined with 95% Confidence Interval (CI). All tests were two tailed. The entire analyses were performed using STATA, Version 16.0 (Stata Corp., College Station, TX, USA).

Results

With respect to the last week in April 2020, the cumulative incidence remains to be flattened in DE, with the confirmed SARS-CoV2, $n = 4,575$ (47.5 per 10,000), Sussex County, $n = 2,114$ (111.4 per 10,000), Kent County, $n = 728$ (41.8 per 10,000) and New Castle County, $n = 1,701$ (28.7 per 10,000). Although not in the table, throughout the state, SARS-CoV2 case positivity was higher among females, $n = 2,456$ (54%) relative to males, $n = 2,083$ (46%).

SARS-CoV2 Case Positivity (Seropositivity) by County

Table 28.1 illustrates the cumulative incidence (CmI) of SARS-CoV2 case positivity rate per 10,000 in DE by county during the last week of April 2020. The rate was highest in Sussex County, 2.3 per 10,000, intermediate in Kent County, 1.7 per 10,000 and lowest in New Castle County, 1.2 per 10,000. While the rate in the state of DE was, 1.8 per 10,000, Sussex County reflected the epicenter of SARS-CoV2 transmission in the state (1.8 vs 2.3 per 10,000).

Table 28.2 demonstrates the cumulative incidence (CmI) of SARS-CoV2 positivity during the first week of May 2020. Figure 28.1 visualizes SARS-CoV2 case positivity rate per 10,000 during April, May and November, 2020, by county. Regardless of the geographic locale and the time period, positive linear trends were observed.

SARS-CoV2 Cumulative Incidence by Race/Ethnicity

The cumulative incidence (CmI) during April, 2020 was highest for non-Hispanic Blacks (NHB) 27% ($n = 1250$), intermediate among non-Hispanic Whites (NHW), $n = 1145$ (25%) and

Table 28.1 Cumulative Incidence and Mortality of COVID-19, Stratified by County, State of Delaware, April, Last Week, 2020

Geographic locale	Confirmed cases (+ve)	Rate per 10,000	Mortality	Rate per 10,000
	Number (%)		Number (%)	
New Castle (North)	1,903 (36.5)	34.1	65 (36.7)	1.16
Kent (Mid-Central)	821 (15.8)	15.5	30 (16.9)	1.66
Sussex (South)	2,461 (42.3)	105.1	55 (30.1)	2.26
Delaware State	5,208	53.5	177	1.80

Notes, abbreviations and Data Source: The rates were computed based on the US Census population size of DE and the counties based on the 2018 projection. DE population, $n = 973,764$, New Castle County, $n = 558,753$, Kent County, $n = 180,786$ and Sussex County, $n = 234,225$.
Data Source: Delaware Department of Health and Social Services (DHSS).

Table 28.2 Cumulative Incidence and Mortality of COVID-19, Stratified by County, State of Delaware, May, First Week, 2020

Geographic locale	Confirmed cases (+ve)	Rate per 10,000	Mortality	Rate per 10,000
	Number (%)		Number (%)	
New Castle (North)	1,979 (36.8)	33.5	70 (44.3)	1.25
Kent (Mid-Central)	847 (16.3)	48.6	30 (19.0)	1.66
Sussex (South)	2,520 (46.9)	132.3	58 (36.7)	2.50
Delaware State	5,371	55.8	—	1.80

Notes and abbreviation: There were 25 cases without county identification. The rates were computed based on the US Census population size of DE and the counties based on the 2018 projection. Delaware State (DE) population, n = 973,764, New Castle County, n = 558,753, Kent County, n = 180,786 and Sussex County, n = 234,225.
Data Source: Delaware Department of Health and Social Services (DHSS).

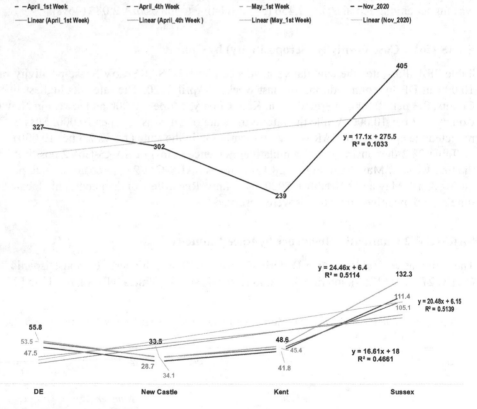

Figure 28.1 SARS-CoV2 Case Positivity Rate (per 10,000) in Delaware, Stratified by County, April–May, November, 2020

Notes, abbreviations and Data Source: R^2 = Coefficient of determination, implying the contributory effect of X (independent variable) to Y (response or dependent variable). DE = State of Delaware, USA.
Data Source: Delaware Department of Health and Social Services (DHSS).

Hispanics, n = 865 (19%) but lowest among multiracial, n = 234 (5%) and Asian/Pacific Islanders, n = 61 (1%). The unidentified race CmI was relatively higher, n = 1020 (22%). Most confirmed cases in Hispanics were in Sussex County, n = 628 (30%), while most confirmed cases for NHB and NHW were in New Castle County, n = 678 (41%) and n = 556 (33%), respectively.

SARS-CoV2 Case Positivity Rate by Race/Ethnicity Stratified by County

Although not on the table, there were racial and geo-clustering differentials in cumulative incidence of SARS-CoV2. The rate was highest among Hispanics in Sussex County, 479.5 per 10,000. With respect to New Castle County, the rate was highest among Hispanics, 145.6 per 10,000, intermediate among NHB, 72.7 per 10,000 and lowest among NHW, 21.6 per 10,000. Regarding Kent County, the rate was highest among Hispanics, 91.1 per 10,000, intermediate among NHB, 21.8 per 10,000 and NHW, 22.2 per 10,000. (Figure 28.2) shows the SARS-CoV2 case positivity by race/ethnicity and geographic locale as geo-coding or geo-clustering. The Sussex County, the south of DE exhibits excess case positivity relative to the state and other counties.

During April, the disproportionate burden of SARS-CoV2 among Hispanics in DE was 100.2 per 10,000, with the highest burden among Hispanics in Sussex County, 313.0 per 10,000, while this was intermediate among NHB in DE, 59.6 per 10,000 and was similar in terms of geo-clustering to Hispanics in Sussex County, NHB, 104.5 per 10,000. Whereas the population size of Hispanics is 9.3% in DE, this population represents an estimated 19% of SARS-CoV2 case positivity, implying 2.04 times as likely for Hispanics to be positive for SARS-CoV2, relative to its population contribution.

Similarly, while NHB constitutes 21.5% of the total population of DE, a disproportionate burden of SARS-CoV2 case positivity was observed, 1.30, implying a 30% disproportionate burden of this pandemic.

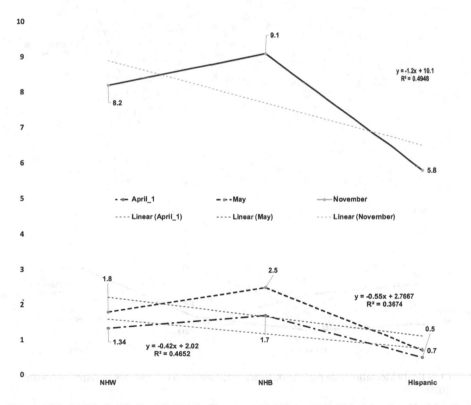

Figure 28.2 SARS-CoV2 Case Positivity Rate per 10,000 by Race/Ethnicity Stratified by County, DE, May 2020

Notes, abbreviations and Data Source: R^2 = Coefficient of determination, implying the contributory effect of X (independent variable) to Y (response or dependent variable). DE = State of Delaware, USA.

Data Source: Delaware Department of Health and Social Services (DHSS).

COVID-19 Case Fatality and Mortality Risk

There were racial/ethnic differentials in the cumulative mortality, and was higher among NHB, 1.70 per 10,000 compared to NHW, 1.34 per 10,000. In terms of univariable binomial modeling of population at risk and the outcome, COVID-19 mortality, NHB relative to NHW were 27% more likely to die from COVID-19, unadjusted risk ratio (uRR) = 1.27, 95% CI, 0.85–1.89, with attributable fraction of the exposed (AFE) = 20.9, 95% CI, −18 to 47.0, and population attributable fraction of 6.0%. (Figure 28.3) demonstrates COVID-19 mortality by race/ethnicity and time period. Regardless of the time period for COVID-19 mortality, NHB indicated excess mortality relative to NHW in DE.

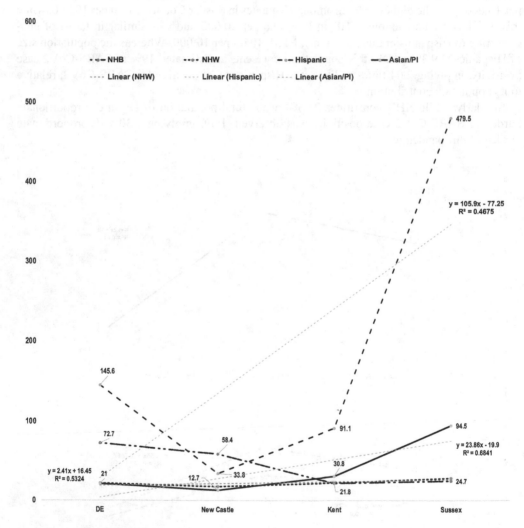

Figure 28.3 COVID-19 Mortality Rate per 10,000 by Race/Ethnicity, in Delaware State, April–November, 2020

Notes, abbreviations and Data Source: R^2 = Coefficient of determination, implying the contributory effect of X (independent variable) to Y (response or dependent variable). DE = State of Delaware, USA.

Data Source: Delaware Department of Health and Social Services (DHSS).

In addition, Figure 28.4 exhibits COVID-19 mortality rate by county and race/ethnicity. With respect to NHB, the mortality rate in the state of DE was higher compared to their NHW counterparts (2.5 per 10,000 vs 1.8 per 10,000). Regardless of the county, the mortality from COVID-19 among NHB was higher relative to their NHW counterparts. In New Castle County the rate was marginally higher among NHB (1.6 per 10,000 vs 1.5 per 10,000). Similarly, in Kent County, there was an increased mortality among NHB relative to NHW (3.3 per 10,000 vs 1.5 per 10,000). Likewise, in Sussex County NHB illustrated excess mortality to NHW (5.9 vs 2.6). In the state of DE as well as all the three counties, mortality was higher among NHB (upper curve) relative to their NHW counterparts.

SARS-CoV2 Case Positivity and COVID-19 Mortality Rate by Selective Zip Codes

Table 28.3 represents the mortality incidence of SARS-CoV2 by geographic locale. With respect to geo-clustering, there was a significant 50% increased risk of dying from COVID-19 in Sussex County compared to the state of DE, incidence rate ratio (IRR) = 1.50, 95% CI, 1.11–2.03. The zip codes with relatively higher mortality were 19720 (New Castle City), 19963

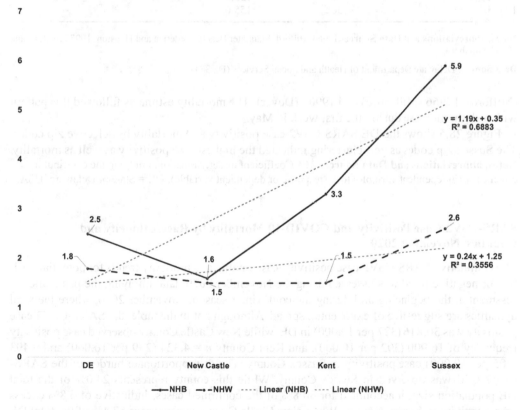

Figure 28.4 State of Delaware (DE) and Counties COVID-19 Mortality Rate per 10,000, stratified by Race/Ethnicity, May 2020

Notes, abbreviations and Data Source: R^2 = Coefficient of determination, implying the contributory effect of X (independent variable) to Y (response or dependent variable). DE = State of Delaware, USA.

Data Source: Delaware Department of Health and Social Services (DHSS).

Table 28.3 COVID-19 Cases Confirmation and Mortality by Geo-Clustering, Delaware Counties

Geo-clustering – zip ode	Confirmed cases (n)	Rate per 10,000	Mortality (n)	Rate per 10,000
New Castle County				
May 5, 2020				
19720	277	42.6	13	2.0
19801	73	46.9	—	—
19805	159	42.5	—	—
19713	104	31.6	—	—
May 6, 2020				
19720	294	45.2	13	2.0
19801	76	48.4	—	—
19805	175	46.4	—	—
19713	113	34.4	—	—
Kent County	891	51.0	33	1.6
Dover/19901	230	67.9	11	2.9
Sussex County	2,764	145.1	75	2.2
19963*	307	141.4	22	6.7
19966	327	139.2	11	2.8
19973	362	155.6	—	—

Notes, abbreviations and Data Source: 19963 Milford, Slaughter Beach, Frederica and Houston. 19973 Seaford and 19963 Millsboro.

Data Source: Delaware Department of Health and Social Services (DHSS).

(Milford), 19966 (Millsboro) and 19901 (Dover). The mortality estimates followed this pattern with a slight increase during the first week in May.

Figure 28.5 shows the DE SARS-CoV2 case positivity and mortality by selective zip codes. The Sussex zip codes as geo-clustering indicated the highest case positivity as well as mortality. **Notes, abbreviations and Data Source**: R^2 = Coefficient of determination, implying the contributory effect of X (independent variable) to Y (response or dependent variable). DE = State of Delaware, USA.

SARS-CoV2 Case Positivity and COVID-19 Mortality by Race/Ethnicity and Counties, November 2020

The cumulative SARS-CoV2 case positivity, case fatality and mortality trends for potential positive or negative trend was assessed using the November 2020 data, implying the pandemic assessment at the beginning and during the cold/winter season, November 2020, where the viral dynamics are suggestive of exponential spread. Although not in the table, the SARS-CoV2 case positivity was 30,816 (327 per 10,000) in DE, while New Castle County observed case positivity frequency of 16,900 (302 per 10,000), and Kent County n = 4,324 (239 per 10,000) and 9,493 (405 per 10,000) case positivity in Sussex County. The disproportionate burden of the SARS-CoV2 CmI was observed in Sussex County. While this county represents 24.0% of the total DE population size, it accounted for 30.8% of the confirmed cases, indicative of 6.8% excess case positivity in Sussex County. While New Castle County accounts for 57.4% of the total DE population size, SARS-CoV2 case positivity was 54.8%, indicative of 2.6% decreased burden of transmission and infectivity in this county. Similarly, there was no disproportionate burden of SARS-CoV2 CmI in Kent County, indicative of 14.0% case positivity, with a population size of 18.6% of the total DE population, implying 4.6% decreased burden of SARS-CoV2 CmI.

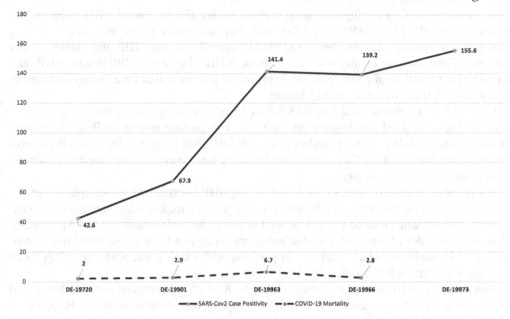

Figure 28.5 Delaware SARS-CoV2 Case Positivity and Mortality Rate per 10,000 by Selected Zip Codes, May 2020

Notes, abbreviations and Data Source: R^2 = Coefficient of determination, implying the contributory effect of X (independent variable) to Y (response or dependent variable). DE = State of Delaware, USA.

Data Source: Delaware Department of Health and Social Services (DHSS).

Although not in the table, the mortality as per November 20, 2020, for the state of Delaware was 746 cases, with a fatality rate of 6.2 per 10,000. The cumulative mortality by race/ethnicity was 492 (66%) for non-Hispanic Whites, 187 (25%) for non-Hispanic Blacks, 52 (7%) for Hispanics, and 12 (2%) for multiracial. NHB illustrate the disproportionate burden of COVID-19 mortality in DE relative to their White counterparts. Specifically, while the population size of NHB is 21.9% as per the US Census 2018 data, mortality was 25%, indicative of excess mortality of 3.1% as disproportionate burden of dying from COVID-19 in this population. In contrast, while the population size of NHW is 69.1%, the mortality CmI or period prevalence was 66% indicative of 3.1% decreased burden of COVID-19 mortality among NHW.

Discussion

With the current COVID-19 pandemic, and the US with the highest confirmed cases and mortality globally as well as the disproportionately observed mortality in some subpopulations, there remains an urgent need to examine these data, provide a possible explanation to the observed racial/ethnic disparities and geo-clustering in DE, and propose feasible recommendations in racial/ethnic and geo-clustering or geo-environmental gap narrowing in SARS-CoV2 infectivity and COVID-19 mortality. Aggregate data were utilized from the Delaware Department of Health and Social Services (DHSS) where demographic information was available to determine the racial variances in the confirmed SARS-CoV2 cases and mortality as well as risk differentials, comparing the NHW, NHB and Hispanics subpopulation deaths, as well as geo-variances in CmI case positivity and mortality. There are a few relevant findings to epidemic curve flattening and case fatality mitigation in communities of color, namely NHB, Hispanics in Sussex County, DE. First, SARS-CoV2 CmI varied by race, ethnicity, county and sex. Second, there was a disproportionate burden of COVID-19 mortality among NHB and Sussex County residents. Third, the case fatality was higher among NHB relative to NHW. Fourth, NHB relative to NHW regardless of geographic locale presented with increased case fatality and mortality risk in COVID-19 in the state of Delaware.

This study has demonstrated that SARS-CoV2 CmI varied by race, ethnicity, geographic locale and sex. The CmI was highest among NHW, intermediate among NHB and Hispanics, but lowest among Asian/Pacific Islanders. However, NHB and Hispanics illustrated the disproportionate burden of SARS-CoV2. Previous literature had observed a comparable pattern of transmission in different settings.[7]

The observed burden of SARS-CoV2 CmI among NHB is explained by workplace segregation, where NHB are employed in jobs with fewer or no benefits, but with more adverse conditions, such as buildings with no fire exit, as well as a stressful environment in DE.[13] Specifically, NHB and Hispanics who are employed as public transit drivers have an increased risk of contracting viral microbes, which explains, in part, the SARS-CoV2 infectivity and COVID-19 mortality racial/ethnic burden differentials.

This study has also observed an increase in the SARS-CoV2 disproportionate burden of CmI among residents of Sussex County as well as the disproportionate burden among Hispanics in this county. The observed geo-clustering is due to the increasing population density of Hispanics in this county as well as the type of employment which predisposed this subpopulation to increased exposure to such environments with exponential viral spread, mainly meat factory workers, sanitation jobs, maids, and restaurant and hotel housekeeping.[14,15,16] In addition, the workplace segregation as well as uncompensated sick time may explain, in part, the excess SARS-CoV2 transmission among Hispanics in this county.

The current study clearly observed higher case fatality among NHB relative to NHW. Previous studies of the flu pandemics of 1918 and 2009 clearly implicated the socially disadvantaged individuals and populations in survival disadvantage following infectivity.[7] The excess case fatality among NHB is explained in part by the higher prevalence of chronic diseases, namely hypertension and other cardiovascular diseases, diabetes and cancer, as well as aberrant epigenomic modulation in COVID-19 prognosis and mortality.[7] NHB are more likely, compared to their NHW counterparts, to be diagnosed with type II diabetes, primary HTN, stroke and malignant neoplasm and have higher mortality from these conditions.[17,18] The higher incidence of these conditions among NHB has been associated with a lack of access to healthcare as well as decreased healthcare utilization due to several obstacles and barriers.[18]

Second, the social determinants of health (SDH), which reflect the needed resources to benefit from optimal health outcomes, are not equitably available for NHB.[17,18] These determinants are characterized by the social gradient as lower social hierarchy, upon which the socially disadvantaged individuals or populations are less likely to benefit from early education, quality education through college and a well-paying job. The SDH, namely education, socioeconomic status, income, employment, food security, racism, safe environment, insurance, transportation and living conditions, adversely impact morbidity and mortality outcomes among NHB in the US.[19,20,21]

Since NHBs are predisposed to more environmental pollutants and toxins, psychosocial stressors, a dangerous job environment and incarceration, these environments interact with the gene, implying impaired gene expression and increased disease development, poorer prognosis, increased mortality and survival disadvantage. In addition, because social gradient reflects environmental neighborhood characteristics, the understanding of gene and environment interaction, such as living conditions, may provide an additional strategic approach in intervention mapping for disease management and prevention. In effect, examining the gene and environment interaction, observed as epigenomics, will provide substantial data on intervention in narrowing the gap between NHB and NHW in DE with respect to COVID-19 mortality.

The gene and environment interaction as epigenomic modulations that commence at gametogenesis are transgenerational but reversible. The social signal transduction that is evoked from the stress placed on NHB and Hispanics has a substantial effect on the sympathetic nervous system and provokes beta-adrenergic receptors. This response has been shown to involve the Conserved Transcriptional Response to Adversity (CTRA) gene expression and the consequent elaboration of pro-inflammatory cytokines, due to impaired gene expression of the transcription factors and the inhibition of gene expression with respect to anti-inflammatory responses.[22] In understanding these pathways of genomic stability and their role in disease causation as well as mortality, epigenomic studies are necessary in determining whether or not Blacks, relative to Whites, have an increased mean deoxyribonucleic acid (DNA) methylation index with respect to the genome-wide analysis. Such an initiative will involve the utilization of the bisulfite pyrosequencing that is very specific in differentiating between the methyl group (CH_3) and hydroxyethyl group, as well as the binding of these groups to the Cytosine-phosphate-Guanine (CpG) non-coding region of the gene, inhibiting transcription and messenger ribonucleic acid (mRNA) sequencing, leading to impaired gene expression and abnormal cellular functionality. The reference to epigenomics investigation reflects the inability of a COVID-19 case to respond to treatment modalities due to the drug receptors unavailability, resulting from impaired gene expression (mRNA translation dysregulation) reflecting a decreased response to COVID-19 treatment among racial/ethnic minorities, namely NHB and Hispanics.[23] The observed aberration epigenomic modulation clearly illustrates treatment effect heterogeneity in which some subpopulations respond differently to a given therapeutic agent in the phase of epigenomic lesion, explaining, in part, racial risk differentials in COVID-19 case fatality.

Despite the rigorous methodology utilized in this racial/ethnic and geo-clustering model for SARS-CoV2 and COVID-19, there are some limitations. First this study utilized pre-existing data as secondary data which are subject to information, selection and misclassification biases. However, the observed disproportionate burden of SARS-CoV2 CmI among NHB and Sussex County in DE is not driven solely by these biases. Second, since risks do not occur in isolation, requiring the application of an explanatory model, namely confounding adjustment, it is unlikely that the predictive mortality risk in this study, which implicated increased COVID-19 mortality and case fatality among NHB and Hispanics in Sussex County, is driven solely by unmeasured confounders.[24]

Conclusion and Recommendations

The Delaware SARS-CoV2 case positivity indicates a disproportionate burden on the communities of color, namely NHB and Hispanics as well as case geo-clustering disproportionate burden in Sussex County, while COVID-19 increased case fatality and mortality was observed among NHB and Sussex County residents. In addition, there was a positive trend in SARS-CoV2 transmission as well as comparable case fatality and mortality risk characterization by race/ethnicity and geo-clustering in the state of DE comparing the initial period of the pandemic with the cold/flu season, 2020. These findings are indicative of the requirement to examine subpopulation needs, namely, NHB and Hispanics for intervention mapping for SARS-CoV2 risk reduction and racial/ethnic as well as county mortality gap narrowing from COVID-19.

These findings indicate the following recommendations in DE COVID-19 case and mortality marginalization by race/ethnicity and geo-clustering:

(1) Based on these data there is an urgent and increasing need for adherence to preventive and control measures in these subpopulations at risk for transmission reduction, mainly Hispanics, NHB and Sussex County residents, including testing, contact tracing, tracking, social and physical distancing as well as non-surgical and non-medical face mask utilization while outside home.

(2) Further, these findings are suggestive of the need to examine the social gradient that may be associated with the disproportionate burden of mortality among NHB as well as an explanation for the increased risk of transmission among Hispanics, especially in Sussex County.

Specifically, the application of these recommendations will enhance the state of DE in curve flattening and down drifting as well as case fatality mitigation, especially among the marginalized and most vulnerable populations. In effect, the second wave is inevitable unless the state successfully implements all the measures recommended for spread mitigation, based on the ongoing scientific data on pandemics. Since health equity is essential in subpopulations risk and health outcomes marginalization, this study clearly recommends that the state of Delaware, through its counties, utilize disproportionate benefit for NHB, Hispanics and Sussex County residents for equitable outcome of SARS-CoV2 transmission and COVID-19 case fatality and mortality.

In future, these data request adherence to viral control and preventive measures, namely: (a) social and physical distancing until the epidemic curve is flattened in DE prior to return to normal economic life, will prevent a significant resurgence of COVID-19 with altered SARS-CoV2 antigenicity or different serotypes. (b) Face mask application throughout the state, especially among COVID-19 positives and symptomatic individuals to marginalize the spread of the virus. (c) The immune system potentiation by providing equitable resources namely balanced lifestyle to food material to Blacks/AA and Hispanics who are socially disadvantaged with low SES in DE, especially those in Sussex County. (d) The education of the NHB and Hispanic communities on the health consequence of COVID-19 through ePublicHealth [B12 session via zoom] Intervention program and the provision of assistance and encouragement for testing, case identification and isolation, will flatten the epidemic curve in the Black communities influencing epidemic curve flattening and down drifting in the epidemic curve nationally, thus enhancing the overall US economy and return to normal lifestyle and coping. This initiative will not only reduce social inequities but the social inequities burden for future diseases and pandemics. (e) Since the disproportionate burden of pandemics fundamentally reflects health disparities, addressing this disproportionate burden in future epidemics and pandemics will require subpopulations, especially NHB, American Indians/Alaska Natives and Hispanics to be provided with the resources necessary for optimal health. Therefore, adherence to the World Health Organization's recommendation of social justice and peace as conditions necessary for health is essential in narrowing health disparities in pandemics by addressing social injustice and systemic and structural racism, thus transforming health equity. The State of Delaware through the Centers for Disease Control and Prevention (CDC) and the DHSS to increase testing throughout the state, especially in the most vulnerable COVID-19 population, namely NHB and Hispanics in Sussex County. (f) The development of surveillance and monitoring systems for data availability on the social determinants of health and race/ethnicity in transforming pandemic health equity is essential in intervention mapping in marginalizing the COVID-19 outcomes among the communities of color. (g) Establishment and implementation of a rapid health equity transformation taskforce and evaluation matrix for risk mitigation among racial and ethnic minorities, namely Blacks/AA and Hispanics. (h) The state, county and local health departments collect socio-demographic data for a better understanding of exposures and confounding in viral spread and case fatality. (i) As we anticipate the mRNA vaccine for SARS-CoV2 host "spike" protein generation for antibody production, the administration of this novel technology vaccine must be initiated among the most vulnerable populations, especially the socially disadvantaged population, namely NHB and Hispanics for herd immunity in these subpopulations prior to other communities' immunizations.

Further, as an epidemiologic perspective, these data recommend emergency preparedness in health equity resources through disproportionate universalism, which is the public health lens in the provision of health services more to racial/ethnic minorities before the non-vulnerable populations. The failure to address the socially disadvantaged individuals and populations' needs in our society, namely the state of Delaware, by educational opportunity, equitable employment opportunity and the departure from structural racism, will render the Delawareans more vulnerable to public health and healthcare crises in this pandemic. In effect, as clinicians, researchers, health officers, epidemiologists, infectious disease specialists, and public health experts, it is our moral responsibility regardless of our race/ethnicity, gender or age, to rapidly respond to the disproportionate mortality burden of this pandemic in the communities of color, especially NHB, since human life remains a primary value.

Questions for Discussion

1. What is the research question and hypothesis utilized in this analytic epidemiologic study on SARS-CoV2 and COVID-19?
2. Describe the epidemiologic design utilized in this study and examine the data source.
3. Is this study a primary or secondary data assessment in SARS-CoV2 seropositivity and COVID-19 mortality?
4. What is the statistical analytic method utilized in these data assessment?
5. Are these data ecologic or individual level data? What are the limitations in the utilization of an ecologic data in SARS-CoV2 seropositivity and COVID-19 mortality parameter estimation?
6. What are the main findings in this study and the limitations of this study?
7. Is there confounding assessment in this study, and the inclusion of such variables in a reliable parameter estimate, with respect to the nexus between the independent and outcome variable? Was the effect measure modifier as heterogeneity effect observed in this study?
8. Is the inference or conclusion reliable and accurate?
9. What are the suggestions or recommendation in future research?
10. Are the references appropriately cited?

Notes

1 Anderson RM, Heesterbeek H, Klinkenberg D, Hollingsworth TD. "How Will Country-based Mitigation Measures Influence the Course of the COVID-19 epidemic?" *Lancet* (2020) 395(10228) 931–934. DOI:https://doi.org/10.1016/S0140–6736(20)30567-5.
2 Giwa A and Desai A. (2020). "Novel Coronavirus COVID-19: An Overview for Emergency Clinicians". *Emerg Med Pract* (2020) 22(2 Suppl 2): 1–21.
3 Estreicher M, Hranjec T, Pepe PE. et al. "Spotting the Clotting: Hypercoagulopathy in COVID-19". (2020). Available at: https://www.emsworld.com/1224381/spotting-clottinghypercoagulopathy-covid-19. Accessed 20 Nov. 2020

4 Bikdeli B, Madhavan MV, Jimenez D, Chuich T, Dreyfus I, Driggin E et al. (2020). "COVID-19 and Thrombotic or Thromboembolic Disease: Implications for Prevention, Antithrombotic Therapy, and Follow-up". *J Am Coll Cardiol* (2020) 75(23) [epub ahead of print]. doi:10.1016/j.jacc.2020.04.031.

5 Omran AR. "The Epidemiologic Transition: A Theory of the Epidemiology of Population Change. 1971". *The Milbank Quarterly* (2005) 83(4): 731–757. https://doi.org/10.1111/j.1468- 0009.2005.00398.

6 McKeown RE. (2009). "The Epidemiologic Transition: Changing Patterns of Mortality and Population Dynamics". *American Journal of Lifestyle Medicine* (2009) 3(1 Suppl): 19S–26S. https://doi.org/10.1177/1559827609335350462.

7 Holmes Jr, L, Enwere E, Williams J, Ogundele B, Chavan P, et al. (2020). "Black–White Risk Differentials in COVID-19 (SARS-CoV-2) Transmission, Mortality and Case Fatality in the United States: Translational Epidemiologic Perspective and Challenges". *Int J Environ Res* (2020) 17(2): 4322 doi:10.3390/ijerph17124322.

8 Rothe C, Schunk M, Sothmann P et al. "Transmission of 2019-nCoV Infection from an Asymptomatic Contact in Germany". *N Engl J Med* (2020) 382(10): 970–971. doi:10.1056/NEJMc2001468.

9 Singhal T. "A Review of Coronavirus Disease-2019 (COVID-19)". *Indian Journal of Pediatrics* (2020) 87(4): 281–286. https://doi.org/10.1007/s12098-020-03263-6.

10 Mohanty SK, Satapathy A, Naidu MM, Mukhopadhyay S, Sharma S, Barton LM, Stroberg E, Duval EJ, Pradhan D, Tzankov A, Parwani AV. "Severe Acute Respiratory Syndrome Coronavirus-2 (SARS-CoV-2) and Coronavirus Disease 19 (COVID-19) – Anatomic Pathology Perspective on Current Knowledge". *Diagnostic Pathology* (2020) 15(1): 103. https://doi.org/10.1186/s13000-020-01017–8476.

11 Holmes Jr, L. "Applied Epidemiologic Principles and Concept: Clinician's Guidelines to Study Conduct and Interpretation, CRC". (2018). Available at: https://www.routledge.com/Applied- Epidemiologic-Principles-and-Concepts-Clinicians-Guide-to-Study/Jr/p/book/9780367560089479. Accessed 18 Nov. 2020.

12 DHSS, Delaware Health and Social Services. "My Healthy Community: Delaware Environmental Public Health Tracking Network". Available at: https://myhealthycommunity.dhss.delaware.gov/locations/state. Accessed 21 Nov. 2020.

13 Gee GC and Ford CL. (2011). "Structural Racism and Health Inequities: Old Issues, New Directions". *Du Bois Review: Social Science Research on Race* (2011) 8(1): 115–132. https://doi.org/10.1017/S1742058X11000130486.

14 Krogstad JM, Gonzalez-Barrera A, Lopez MH. "Hispanics More Likely than Americans Overall to See Coronavirus as a Major Threat to Health and Finances". (2020). Pew Research Center. Available at: https://www.pewresearch.org/fact-tank/2020/03/24/hispanics-more-likely- than-americans-overall-to-see-coronavirus-as-a-major-threat-to-health-and-finances/. Accessed 20 Nov. 2020.

15 Despres C. "Coronavirus Case Rates and Death Rates for Latinos in the United States. Salud America!" (2020). Available at: https://salud-america.org/coronavirus-case-rates-and-death-rates-for-latinos-in-the-united-states/. Accessed 20 Nov. 2020.

16 CDC, Centers for Disease Control and Prevention. "National Center for Health Statistics. Weekly Updates by Select Demographic and Geographic Characteristics. Provisional Death Counts for Coronavirus Disease (COVID-19)". (2020). Available at: https://www.cdc.gov/nchs/nvss/vsrr/covid_weekly/. Accessed Nov. 22, 2020.

17 Lincoln KD, Abdou CM, Lloyd D. "Race and Socioeconomic Differences in Obesity and Depression among Black and non-Hispanic White Americans". *Journal of Health Care for the Poor and Underserved* (2014) 25(1): 257–275. https://doi.org/10.1353/hpu.2014.0038.

18 NASEM, National Academies of Sciences, Engineering, and Medicine; Health and Medicine Division; Board on Population Health and Public Health Practice; Committee on Community-Based Solutions to Promote Health Equity in the United States; Baciu A, Negussie Y, Geller A et al., editors. *Communities in Action: Pathways to Health Equity*. Washington (DC): National Academies Press (US); 2017 Jan 11. 2, "The State of Health Disparities in the United States". Available from: https://www.ncbi.nlm.nih.gov/books/NBK425844/. Accessed 8 Nov. 2020.

19 Singh, GK, Daus GP, Allender M, Ramey CT, Martin E.K, Perry C, Reyes A, Vedamuthu IP. (2017). "Social Determinants of Health in the United States: Addressing Major Health Inequality Trends for the Nation, 1935–2016". *International Journal of MCH and AIDS* (2017) 6(2): 139–164. https://doi.org/10.21106/ijma.236.

20 Walker RJ, Strom Williams J, Egede LE. "Influence of Race, Ethnicity and Social Determinants of Health on Diabetes Outcomes". *The American Journal of the Medical Sciences* (2016) 351(4): 366–373. https://doi.org/10.1016/j.amjms.2016.01.008.

21 Noonan AS, Velasco-Mondragon HE, Wagner FA. "Improving the Health of African Americans in the USA: An Overdue Opportunity for Social Justice". *Public Health Rev* (2016) 37: 12. https://doi.org/10.1186/s40985-016-0025-4.

22 Holmes L Jr, Shutman E, Chinaka C, Deepika K, Pelaez L, Dabney KW. (2019). "Aberrant Epigenomic Modulation of Glucocorticoid Receptor Gene (NR3C1) in Early Life Stress and Major Depressive Disorder Correlation: Systematic Review and Quantitative Evidence Synthesis". *International Journal of Environmental Research and Public Health* (2019) 16(21): 4280. https://doi.org/10.3390/ijerph16214280.

23 Sanders JM, Monogue ML, Jodlowski TZ, Cutrell JB et al. "Pharmacologic Treatments for Coronavirus Disease 2019 (COVID-19): A Review". *JAMA* (2020) 323(18): 1824–1836. doi:10.1001/jama.2020.6019.

24 Holmes L, Chan W, Jiang Z et al. (2007). "Effectiveness of Androgen Deprivation Therapy in Prolonging Survival of Older Men Treated for Locoregional Prostate Cancer". *Prostate Cancer Prostatic Dis* (2007) 10: 388–395. https://doi.org/10.1038/sj.pcan.4500973.

Index

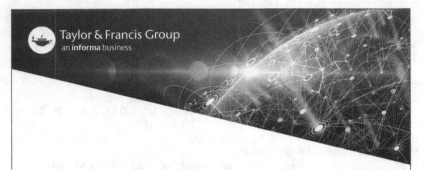

Printed in the United States
by Baker & Taylor Publisher Services

Printed in the United States
by Baker & Taylor Publisher Services